WE ARE WHAT WE LISTEN TO

The Impact of **music** on individual and social **health**

PATRICIA **CAICEDO**
M.D., PH.D.

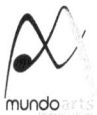

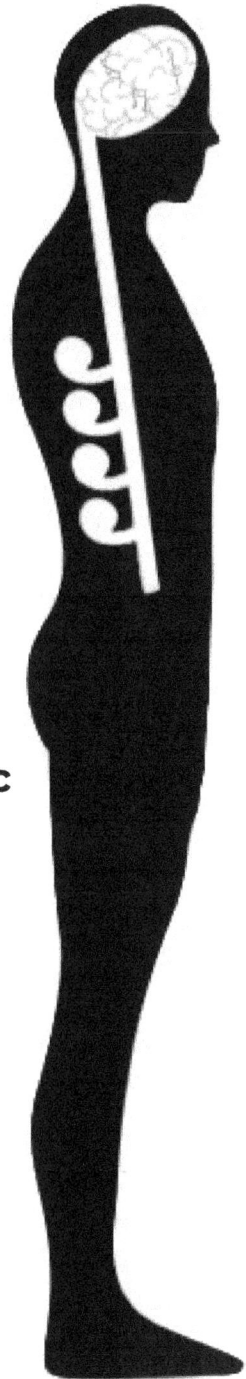

mundoarts

Music and Health Collection N.1
We are what we listen to: the impact of music on individual and social health

ISBN 978-1-7378920-1-4
Hard Cover
October, 2021
MA00012

First edition in Spanish:
Somos lo que escuchamos: impacto de la música en la salud individual y social. Barcelona, Septiembre, 2021

English translation
Neha Iyer

Cover Design
Stephannie Vega
Patricia Caicedo

Interior Design
Patricia Caicedo

Mundo Arts Publications
Patricia Caicedo

www.mundoarts.com

E-mail: **info@mundoarts.com**
Phone US: +1-678-608-3588
Phone Spain: +34-696-144-766

Barcelona - New York

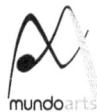

WE ARE
WHAT WE
LISTEN
TO The Impact of **music** on individual and social **health**

PATRICIA **CAICEDO**
M.D., PH.D.

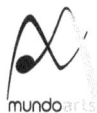

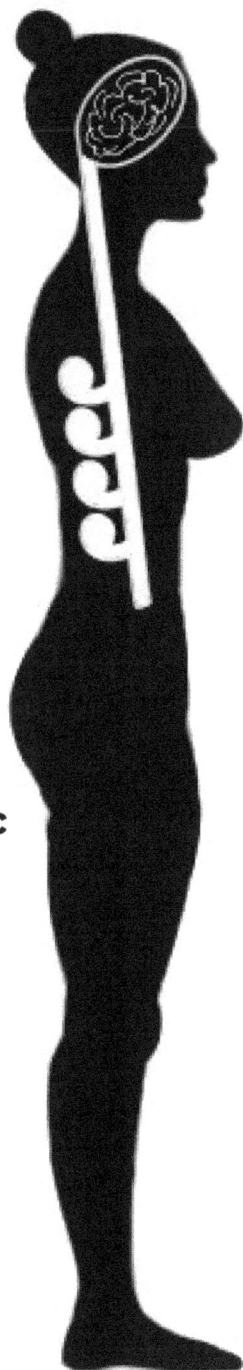

mundoarts

*To my parents Jorge and Patricia
and my brother Juan Pablo.*

INDEX

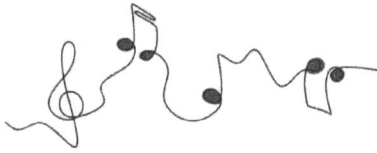

FOREWORD

By Tess Knigthton, Ph.D.

What is the soundtrack of your life? Which music gives you goosebumps? How can a song, like Proust's proverbial *madelaine* dipped in lime-blossom tea, effortlessly and involuntarily, bring back a hundred memories? Have you thought about which music attracts you and why? Do you lose yourself in music or listen to it with a conscious desire to understand it? Or both, depending on circumstances, on the moment in time? How is it that music seems to be able to express our deepest emotions without need for words? Can we ever really know how music works its magic? These are just some of the questions posed by the singer and musicologist Patricia Caicedo in her new book *We are what we listen to.*

Music holds meaning for us, she argues, for each of us as an individual, and for all of us collectively, as a community of the world. That meaning may be influenced – even conditioned – by social and cultural context, but we all participate in 'musicking', the term coined by Christopher Small to indicate that each musical act is experienced by all those present, whether as performer or ear-witness. Music is quintessentially inclusive, even when it may appear to be exclusive, a music with which we are not familiar, a music that can make us feel uneasy even as it draws us to it, a music associated with a particular social group that we do not immediately identify as ours. Music can transcend all barriers, if we allow it to do so. And in this – and many other respects – music is wonderful in its effects – its impact – on our daily life, filling us with wonder at its power, its creative energy, its unswerving companionship from before we are born until after we die, as – often unwittingly – we write our musical autobiography in the course of our lived experience.

Caicedo's book is itself a wonderful introduction to thinking about how music is an integral part of our lives, because, as she describes, it is good for us. During my childhood in England, there was a country saying 'An apple a day keeps the doctor away', and some parents, including my own, would take this quite literally – at least during the apple season. Caicedo, as a trained medical doctor who was known in the hospital where she worked as 'the singing doctor', would say – or, rather sing – 'A song a day keeps the doctor away', and it is an enlightening combination of medical knowledge and musical experience that she brings to this brief survey of, essentially, how music *works*. It is a book that you will want to devour in one sitting (we are what we eat!), but it is filled with ideas that you will want to savour, and with ideas that may take a little while to digest. Music, she argues, is a biological, chemical and psychological process: our physiological, rational and emotional responses are inextricably bound together, even though science is able to detect and chart these responses with increasing accuracy and an unprecedented rapidity with each technological advance. The discovery that our biological cells actually emit sound – they sing! –, that a rich chemical cocktail is mixed inside us when we 'musick', and that the parts of our brain that light up in response to both environmental and organised sound connect to memory and enhance a sense of interconnectedness within ourselves and with others, certainly gives pause for thought.

Caicedo, as doctor and performer, explains these complex processes with clinical clarity and draws on her own experience to elucidate what they mean in practice: how we can listen to our body – our pulse, our rate of breathing, our sense of physical equilibrium – through listening to music; and how we can take stock of our mental well-being by allowing ourselves to enter into the flow of the music and engage with the now of life, emerging able to face the future, to look back at the past without being in thrall to it, and to make the most of the present. Should we, then, regard music as a panacea for all ills? Studies show that 'musicking' can alleviate pain, can reduce sickness from radiotherapy, can prolong life or at least mitigate the aging process, can release emotional tension and restore mental equilibrium, though probably not to the same extent in all people, nor in all situations. A lively debate followed the piping of Classical music in certain stations of the Paris *métro* with the idea of reducing crime. The move appeared to be remarkably effective, until it became apparent that the crimewave itself just moved to other stations where Bach and Beethoven were not to be heard. Did the experiment prove that Classical music had a salutary effect on the criminal mind, or were the criminals deterred simply by their sense of musical taste?

The positive impact of music has been charted by writers from ancient times to the present day, and Caicedo cites many authorities from the past three thousand years and more, from western and eastern traditions. Observation on how music can assuage the sadness and grief felt at the death of a loved one, often leading to a sense of catharsis by which loss is gradually transformed into memory and acceptance, or how it can arouse a sense of exhilaration among a crowd that results in a wave of emotion contagion, as at a spectacular event, whether in coliseum or football stadium, is not new, but reappears in different modes of expression over the centuries. Caicedo's writing is refreshingly free of jargon; it is aware of present-day sensibilities, but wokeness is, thankfully, absent. The book is thoughtful and will make you think; it is affirmative, but grounded in real experience rather than the chimera of fantasy. The reader is drawn into a shared soundscape that is constantly in a state of flux and reflux and in which music is both constant and ever-changing.

Caicedo is surely right to conclude that the role of music in our lives has become even more important in the time of a pandemic, even when live performance has been for almost two years confined to Zoom and podcasts. The ban on singing in choirs has been particularly destructive in terms of sociability and the sheer joy of participating in music-making in the company of others. This is something that many of us have experienced and still miss in a masked, distanced and confined world. But what I didn't know, before reading this wonderful book, is that singing in groups strengthens the presence of oxytocin in the body, a hormone that is released naturally at childbirth to stimulate bonding between mother and child. We may all have sensed that music is a catalyst that can bring elements together and transform them, but it now appears that our sixth sense can be confirmed by a bodily chemical reaction.

This need not take the mystery out of music-making. The fifteenth-century philosopher – and medical doctor – Marsilio Ficino (one of the many authors cited by Caicedo) wonderfully evoked this mystery – or magic, as Caicedo calls it – by describing music as the 'decoration of silence': an increasingly poignant metaphor in an age of unprecedented sound contamination. Ficino, and other thinkers of the time, saw the role of the performer as someone with the ability to channel higher creative activity: performance was considered, essentially, to be a ritual that could create the conditions for contemplative awareness. For them, as for Caicedo, the energy generated by music can be gathered and sustained through the performer, who serves as conduit during the unfolding of the musical performance in an infinite exchange of ebb and flow with the listener. It is this intangible dialogue that can lead to that frisson of understanding, of recognition of all that is beauty, all that is positive, all that is health-giving – and which gives us the goosebumps.

Tess Knighton, ICREA Research Professor
Universitat Autònoma de Barcelona

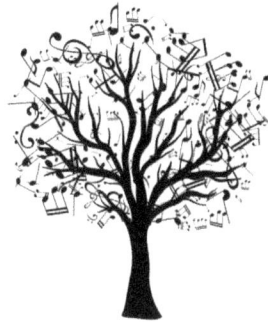

PRELUDE

I'm sure you can think of pieces of music which have defined the most important moments of your life, songs which have been there for you in difficult times, which have helped you express your emotions in a way like no other. Perhaps you have felt an uncontrollable energy after attending a huge concert, an inner peace while listening to a symphony or the desire to cry while listening to a love song.

The fact is that all of us, no matter the time or our culture, have experienced the power of sound, vibration and music.

In the Kybalion,[1] a compilation of texts from Ancient Egypt, published in 1908, we find the seven principles that rule the universe, one of which states: *Nothing is immobile, everything moves, everything vibrates.*[2] This supposedly simple affirmation has been validated right from quantum physics, resulting in string theory which explains how the universe and all its objects function in terms of vibrations of thin supersymmetric strings that move in ten dimensions space-time and one temporary dimension.

The universe is a symphony of objects in constant vibration, life itself is vibration, sound. For example, as proven recently by Pelling, Gralla and Gimzewski,[3] the cells in our body sing, and their song varies depending on health and sickness.

According to my parents, my relationship with music began in my mother's womb, when, very ahead of their time, they played music hoping that it would have a positive effect on my brain development. At five years old, I began my studies in the conservatory, immersing myself in the universe of sounds and finding my most loyal partner in music, my refuge in difficult times and my therapeutic, cathartic tool.

Just like for you, in my own life, music has played different roles, all of which have been of vast importance. When I was eleven years old, when I began to sing, music helped me with social integration, something which was very difficult for me considering I was a profoundly shy child. Singing became my way of expressing emotions, and helped me fit into a group in school, something which I would never have been able to do without it. During my adolescence, it became key to the construction of my identity, a symbol of rebellion, a vehicle of values and ideologies. If I take a look back at my life, music has been present in the most important moments of my life, the celebrations, the sorrows, the loves or the heartbreaks.

Medicine entered my life when I was sixteen, and I began a degree in the Colombian School of Medicine. I remember that the first thing I did when I arrived at the faculty was look for the college choir. Once again, music became the key which opened all doors. Throughout my years at university, I took part in the choir, where I met some of my best friends. When I began clinical practice, in every hospital I was in, I performed concerts for patients and doctors, raising funds for the many hospital services, even becoming known as "the doctor who sings".

I've always known, intuitively so, that music had a healing effect, that patients who listened to it felt better, that even for a few moments, their pain was eased, that they felt happier and more relaxed, which was a feeling also shared by the doctors in the hospital environment, a very demanding environment from a physical and psychological viewpoint.

However, it was only a few years later that I could myself confirm the therapeutic power of music, when the study of singing and the discipline associated with it, which consists of breathing, posture, body consciousness and sound, cured me of an eating disorder that I sustained for many years. It was through music that I became healthy, and learned to listen to myself, even realising that my mental and physical health depended on musical practice, which was the moment I decided to dedicate myself professionally to music and do a complete 180 degree turn in my life.

Although in that moment it felt like I had abandoned medicine, when I began my role as a singing teacher, I realised that every lesson was like a therapeutic session, a medical session where we worked on psychological conflicts and physical pains, and we relearnt how to sense and express using the body and emotions, all through the medium of sound.

I was able to confirm that the journey to health and wellbeing is made up of the conscious composition of a harmonious piece of music, unique to each person and each object in this universe. This piece must also be rhythmic because the universe, as highlighted by the Ancient Egyptians, is also rhythm.

Everything in the universe has its own sound and its own rhythm, the heart and even Covid-19, which, while I'm currently writing this book, is devastating the planet. While I am writing these lines, I am listening to the decoded melody by professor Markus Buehler from MIT, who, along with his team, assigned each aminoacid, the building blocks of protein, a unique note, which then an algorithm turned into musical notes. According to Buehler, listening to the melody offers a more intuitive form of understanding protein: "I would need many different images, a lot of different magnifications to see what the ear can capture with just a few seconds of music."[4]

Perhaps in the future, this auditory comprehension will be key to understanding many pathologies, which until this day have been difficult to understand and treat. Through sound and music, we can more quickly and directly reach the core of the things which surround us, and understand this universe, in which everything from the most microscopic to the most gigantic of objects vibrates.

This makes sense considering it is through sound that we experience life for the first time. As we are born, we interact with the sounds of the environment, creating emotional ties through the voices, songs, and whispers.

I'm sure that now you are thinking about your own relationship with music, about the role that it has played in your life and your relationships, in the construction of your identity, in your health, or you may even be remembering shared musical experiences that have stayed with you.

Music, apart from being an individual experience of the senses, is also a communal experience with a strong symbolic meaning, a space to represent the values that define our identity. Part of its beauty is that it transcends the sphere of the individual to unite us in a shared experience.

There are so many ways that we could discuss the impact of music at a physical, psychological and social level that I have decided to write this book to try shed light on the important role of music and sound in the human experience, the age-old relationship between music, medicine and health, and the ways in which we perceive and process music at a cerebral level.

This journey into this topic is a reflection of my interdisciplinary training in music, medicine and musicology and for this reason, I'll be looking at historical, social, scientific and musical aspects.

In light of recent neuroscientific research, I aim to explain the cognitive processes of music, to understand how the brain of musicians works and the many benefits of musical practice at a cognitive level, such as protecting the brain and delaying the process of aging.

We will discover the ancient relationship between rhythm, movement and health, the mysterious brain mechanisms that link music, pleasure and emotion, and the many ways in which music improves our quality of life, leads to wellness, happiness and provides us a sense of purpose and meaning in life.

The perception of sound and music, one of the most intimate and personal human experiences, as deep as thought itself, has been key to the evolution of our species and it could also be key to creating an individual who is more conscious of themselves and their surrounding, an individual with a global ecological conscience.

The road to physical, mental and emotional health is sure to be filled with sounds and music. I invite you on this journey so you can start to understand the many ways in which music can change your life for the better.

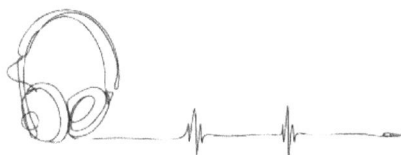

Chapter 1

MUSIC AND MEDICINE
THE HISTORY OF A RELATIONSHIP

Taking shelter in the maternal womb, we begin life floating in a space similar to the sea, in constant movement and vibration. We are accompanied by the rhythmic beat of our mother's heart and the many sounds made by her organs. Upon arriving into the world, a cry is our first mark of independence, an affirmation of *I am*. Gestation and birth are sonorous experiences just like they were for the first hominids hundreds of thousands of years ago. From then on, sound and music have been a central part of human experiences, tools of communication and of healing and above all, spaces of symbolic representation in which our individual and collective identities are built and dealt with.

Because of its ephemeral nature, in that it only exists during the performance, and due to its intangible character, throughout history, music has been associated with magic, spirituality, sublime experiences of the being which transcend the ordinary and transport us to other times, to other states of emotion and consciousness.

Different disciplines, like anthropology, philosophy and archeology have confirmed that music could have preceded the existence of the paleolithic man. Its uses have been as varied as culture itself; right from the origins of humanity, it has been linked to ritual, being a vehicle of ideologies and a social marker.

In his text, *The expression of emotions in animals and man,*[5] published in 1872, Charles Darwin developed the hypothesis that music was necessary for sexual selection, having existed before language itself. Seemingly our Neanderthal ancestors communicated through gestures and vocalizations where they made variations in tone or pace[6].

It is precisely the ability to differentiate the variations of rhythm, tone, timbre and volume in language which allows us to distinguish emotions and the context of a conversation, even in languages that we don't know. It seems that we recognize a primary, very ancient form of communication, based on the musical aspects of communication. According to Daniel Levitin, "humans discovered communication through language, and then, at some point, they rediscovered music."[7]

How did this first human communicate and express himself? What ancestral mysteries were uncovered by this primitive voice?

It was precisely the voice, that first form of contact and uniting bond, a cry which expressed pain, sorrow and joy, which discovered the sounds of the depths of the human soul.

For the current-day man, the voice is the umbilical cord which connects him to the past, the manifestation of life right from the first cry, the affirmation of his presence in the world. The voice, a sound emitted from the body, an inseparable part of it, through orality becomes a space of representation. From the oral sphere, we learn to call out and experience being heard; whatever makes noise gives meaning to the ability to hear.

It is precisely the fact that sound is a part of the body, not just through voice, but also through the multiple sounds made by the organs, in a sort of symphony, perfectly balanced and with the same purpose, which makes it impossible to separate the concepts of music-sound and medicine-health.

The French surgeon René Leriche (1879-1955)

defined health as "life in the silence of organs", suggesting that when we have good health, we are not aware of the existence of our body. When our body is silent, we don't need to give it a second thought. Personally, I believe that health and illness both express themselves through sound. The variations of harmony, frequency and rhythm of these sounds are what differentiates health from illness.

In 2002, professors James Gimzewski and Andrew Pelling from the University of California inaugurated the campus of *sonocytology*,[8] upon having discovered through nanotechnology that cells emit frequencies of sound as they vibrate between themselves; cells sing.[9] This surprising discovery is evidence that life consists of vibration and rhythm and that sound is an integral part of the body and of human experience. It also explains the ancient relationship between music and medicine, two disciplines which at the beginning were related to the supernatural, the spiritual and the magical.

There is numerous evidence about the use of music and sound in magic and religious rituals in which shamans, who were the main interlocutors between gods and men, experts of botany, interpreters of dreams, doctors and mystics, used music to cure and to reach altered states of consciousness. The paleolithic figure of the "masked dancer", also known as "the tiny wizard with a musical bow", found in the caves of *Les Trois Frères*, shows an individual in an upright position, wearing the skin and head of a bison, celebrating a type of dance ritual, accompanied by an object which could be interpreted as a wind instrument or a small musical bow similar to those that are used by some tribes in Africa in the present day[10.]

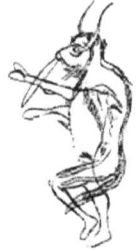

Right from the corners of Siberia to deep in the Amazon, having been a part of the North American and Asian tribes, the shaman has had prominent roles within the community, as a spiritual and social guide, as well as a healer, or medicine-man as it's called in some indigenous tribes.[11] The role of the shaman, undertaken in many cultures by women who were deemed fit to reach out to other realities, was always linked to music and dance, key elements to reach these altered states of consciousness.

Practically all systems of thinking and spiritual traditions have used some type of musical expression to adore, invoke or ask a favor from its deities. Likewise, numerous scientific, religious and philosophical theories, both old and new, credit the structure and existence of the universe to sound.

In Western culture, we usually refer to the *New*

Testament, to the moment when Saint John says: "In the beginning, there was the Word, and the Word was with God, and the Word was God", however, much earlier, around 2000 BC, in old Babylon, in the *Code of Hammurabi,* the Assyrians wrote about the therapeutic use of music in one of the most important documents in history, in which the medical practice is regulated in great detail.[12]

Later on, between the 5th century BC and the 4th century BC, the Ancient Greeks gave great importance to music, considering it an integral part of medicine. Plato stated in *The Republic*, "music is extraordinary because rhythm and harmony make their way to the most intimate part of the soul, and they bestow it with strength and grace". Also, Aristotle studied the effects of music, focusing on its cathartic properties. According to him, music helps "overcome feelings like pity, fear or enthusiasm" and mystic music helps "cure and purify the soul".[13] Both philosophers believed in the healing power of music.

For Pythagoreans, music and mathematics were closely tied. Music, made up of intervals which represent numerical relations, had the same moral attributes as numbers. Their daily routine included playing music in the morning to prepare themselves for their day and night, helping them clear their minds and fall asleep.[14] Pythagoreans also maintained that audible music on the Earth reflected the *Music of the Spheres*.[15]

In his book, *Life of Pythagoras*, Porphyry says:

He himself held morning conferences at his residence, composing his soul with the music of the lute, and singing certain old paeans of Thales. He also sang verses of Homer and Hesiod, which seemed to soothe the mind. He danced certain dances which he conceived conferred on the body agility and health. Walks he took not promiscuously, but only in company of one or two companions, in temples or sacred groves, selecting the quietest and pleasantest places. His friends he loved exceedingly, being the first to declare that the goods of friends are common, and that a friend was another self. While they were in good health he always conversed with them; if they were sick, he nursed them; if they were afflicted in mind, he solaced them, some by incantations and magic charms, others by music. He had prepared songs for the diseases of the body, by the singing of which he cured the sick. He also had some that caused oblivion of sorrow, mitigation of anger and destruction of lust.[16]

Between the 9th and 11th centuries, the Golden Age of Arabic medicine, the famous doctor Ibn Sina (980-1037), author of the *Canon of Medicine*, a book translated into Latin and for centuries considered the reference point for Western doctors, makes special reference to the use of music as therapy. During the Caliphate of Cordoba, mentally ill patients were prescribed a daily dose of listening to beautiful voices and songs[17], and Sufis stated that all of the proceedings of the universe, whether visible or invisible, are musical - we are music. Our bodies vibrate reflecting the symphony of the universe.[18]

While medicine and arts flourished in the Arabic world, in Europe during the Middle Ages, music was an anonymous and collective art, in the same way illness was as well. Together, people suffered the terror, pain and death brought on by successive epidemics, with unknown causes.

When the *Black Death* surfaced, one of the most traumatic events in European history, music and medicine began to have a unexpected association: hoards of men, women and children travelled all over cities and fields dancing frenetically. When the illness began to appear in a city, it wasn't the doctor, but rather the musician to whom they went, believing that only dance would make it disappear. Flagellants, groups of singers, sang songs called *Geisslerlieder*,[19] begging for divine intervention and repenting their sins, and music became like a direct path to God, a tool for healing.

As testament to the relationship between music and medicine during this period came the famous *Decameron*, written not long after bubonic plague which ravaged Florence in 1398. In this, Bocaccio uses ten songs which he wrote in confinement to piece together a story. With the clear purpose of healing, every song is sung in a group as a method of protection against the imminent plague.

So much power was given to music as a healing power that by law, those who wished to be doctors had to appreciate and study music as it was considered essential for maintaining the wellbeing of patients. It was believed that curing the psyche through music also healed the body, and there were even specific melodies recommended for different illnesses. For example, the cure for gout was to listen alternately between the sound of the flute and the harp, but of course, these remedies were only within the reach of a few privileged members of society.

Medical and musical theory are associated with the Hippocrates' four humors - blood, phlegm, yellow bile and black bile - and with the four elements of the cosmos - air, water, land and fire -, stating that both good and bad health depended on the perfect balance between these elements. The pleasure caused by music was clinically prescribed as a remedy for rage, sorrow and fear.

In Italy, Marsilio Ficino (1433-99), physician, musician, astrologer and priest, and one of the most prolific translators of Plato in modern history, wrote in *De vita*[20] (book of life) that music embodies perfection and harmony and induces the feeling of tranquility in its listeners and performers. Ficino also translated the *Song of Orpheus* into Latin, revealing the power of music about nature.[21] According to him, if music is performed with regularity, the spirit adopts the characteristics of the music being listened to. He equated music to the soul, to the intangible, and to the celestial. Like many Renaissance thinkers, he believed illness to be the result of an imbalance of the four humors, in direct relation to nature, so much so that when he treated a patient, he linked their unique nature to the music of the planets.

> "Music is influenced by divine power in such a way that when certain tones are chosen, they reflect the model of the skies and the seven planets. The planets have their own voices and sounds. The sounds of Saturn are slow, profound, jagged and querulous; Mars' are fast, sharp, fierce and threatening; Jupiter has profound and intense, yet always sweet and cheerful harmonies; the music of Venus is voluptuous with a with both wildness and softness, while Apollo's is marked by its grace, reverence

and simplicity, and Mercury's by its vigour and joy".

The Venetian Gioseffo Zarlino (1517-1590), one of the great theorists of Renaissance music, wrote *Istitutioni harmoniche,* a monumental work in which the views of this period of time about the relationship between music and medicine were represented.[22] In his first book, titled *From praise to music*, he states that "absolutely nothing can be found in places where music is not of the greatest interest". According to Zarlino, knowledge of music was essential to be a doctor:

> If the doctor does not understand music, how will he understand the pulse of his patients in the way Herophilus recommended, based on musical proportions?[23]

From 1550 onwards and until the beginning of the 17th century, a lot of effort was put towards elucidating the relationship between music and emotions. It was in *The doctrine of emotions*[24] where the first attempts to link empirical reason with music were expressed, linking science and music to explain the various emotional states like rage, desire, amazement, love, vigor, joy - feelings which, according the theorists at the time, were the opposite of sadness, gentleness and sweetness. This doctrine had a huge influence on Baroque music, as seen in the great works by J.S. Bach or Handel.[25] It is worth noting that during the 17th century, healing arts were represented by Apollo, god of music and medicine.

Important figures at the time brought this topic to the center of their discourse. In 1618, a young René Descartes (1596-1650) published the *Compendium musicae*, in which he explains the pleasure of music using mathematics, which he called the geometry of the senses. In this, he states that music brings pleasure and awakens emotions, giving the sensory organs a predominant role.[26] In 1649, in *Les Passions de l'âme*, he described the six passions in terms of their effects on the mind and their relationship with the movement and spirits of the blood.

In 1650, the German Jesuit, mathematician and philosopher Athanasius Kircher (1601-1680) wrote *Musurgia Universalis*, a piece of work which influenced such important composers as Handel and Bach.[27] In this, he explores the existence of different musical styles and states that the emotional and physiological characteristics of an individual determine their musical preferences in such a way that you can treat a person with different types of music to induce different emotional and physiological states. According to Kircher, the body and soul adopt the spirit of the music.[28]

Up until the 17th century, studies about the relationship between music and health were confined to the intellectual elites of society and although music was used as therapy for many illnesses, it was not known how it worked. The physiological effects of music on health remained a mystery[29] and moreover, music was a phenomenon that occurred in private spaces, to which only a select few had access, and only on special occasions.[30]

It was in the 18th century, accompanied by the Age of the Enlightenment, when texts about music and health became increasingly scientific and focused on understanding the physiological effects of music, including its changes on blood pressure, breathing and digestion.[31] As an example, we can look at the works of *Richard Browne, Medicina musica: or, A mechanical essay on the effects of singing, musick, and dancing, on human bodies* (1727).[32] and those of Richard Brocklesby, *Reflections on Antient [sic] and Modern Musick, with application to the cure of disease* (1749).[33]

Browne begins his book by saying:

"Singing is the enemy of melancholic thoughts, which we are constantly trying to suppress, and therefore singing is a pleasing promoter of mirth and joy. Singing brings serenity of mind, as well as being beneficial for digestion, due to the use of abdominal muscles and the diaphragm. Singing causes muscular elasticity and awakens the mind and body."

Later on, in the 19th century, the German physicist and physician, Hermann von Helmholtz kickstarted the field of acoustic physiology. Considered one of the precursors of experimental psychology, Helmholtz invented the Helmholtz resonator, a piece of apparatus to analyze the combination of tones made by complex natural sounds. His research about the emotional effects of harmonies on the psyche boosted the application of music in a clinical environment and opened the doors to numerous studies in the fields of perception and musicology.

Also in the 19th century, the first use of music therapy in an institutional environment took place on Roosevelt Island (previously named Blackwell Island) in New York, as well as the first systematic experiment of music therapy, in which music was used to alter sleep states during psychotherapy.[34]

In the field of surgery, Dr Evan O'Neill Kane was the first to use music in a surgical environment, and in 1914, he published a report about the use of the phonograph in the operating theatre.[35] The following year, Dr W.P. Burdick published a more detailed description of the experiment in the American Annual of Anaesthesia and Analgesia: "I discovered that patients that listened to music were better able to tolerate the anesthesia and they had a reduced level of anxiety before suffering the "horrors of surgery".[36]

Four decades later, the effect of auditory analgesia was shown while observing a reduced need for painkillers in patients who were undergoing painful dental procedures when exposed to both strong auditory stimulus as well as music in the background. Previous research suggested that being exposed to music reduces haemodynamic variability, postoperative pain, the amount of sedative or painkiller needed and the time of recovery post-operation.[37] It also lowers the levels of dehydroepiandrosterone, epinephrine, interleukin-6 and various other substances associated with stress, and it significantly increases the plasma concentration of the growth hormone, with its subsequent positive impact on immunity.

In the 20th and 21st centuries, new areas of study arose which combined music and medicine, gradually revealing the effects of music, the way in which we process it in the brain and its relationship with our health. We have slowly responded to the questions asked centuries ago and we understand the complex mechanisms that take place in perception of music, not just from a biological point of view but also a cultural one, because although we perceive music through our body, we cannot separate it from its cultural environment. Music is loaded with symbolic content, which reflects the social and cultural values of the context in which it was created.

Although music has an important social role and unquestionable healing powers in all cultures around the world, some people wrongly believe that the only music with therapeutic effects is Western classical music; we remember the famous *Mozart Effect*, which made millions of people believe that listening to the music of Mozart, and only this, made their children more intelligent. This could not be further from the truth. This was so widely believed because of Enlightenment rationalism, which placed Europe at the centre of history and seeped its way into the whole of academia and science, and caused only music coming from Western Europe to be considered legitimate, and therefore the majority of research about the effects of music on health were carried out using this particular type of music.

The truth of the matter is that listening to the music of Mozart positively impacts our health, but luckily it isn't the only music to have this effect. The effect that music has on us is linked to the culture in which we have grown up and the experiences and associations we have with it. The numerous and diverse pieces of music around the world have positive effects on health, on both a physical and emotional level.

Another wonderful aspect of music is that as well as being an individual experience to help us perceive, it is also a collective experience, a way for us to communicate, to fit into a group, to relate to one another. This is why all of us, regardless of the context in which we are born, can identify songs that have marked different periods of our life, that make up, so to speak, our soundtrack, the different moments of our existence. Music therefore has become a social marker and it is linked to emotions, memory and, above all, our identity.

Let's ask ourselves: Why do some songs make us cry, others reawaken our patriotic pride and others transport us to the past? Why do we want to sing some, but we skip others? Why do the same songs change their role and meaning over time, as if they have their own life and write their own story?

Tell me what you listen to and I will brand you with the relevant label. The music that we listen to identifies us and associates us with a set of values, with a class, a place, a generation, a mood, a desire or an aspiration. It speaks about our history, making it the foundation of memory.

It is incredible that a thing so abstract as music is such an integral part of human experience. Its ubiquity and intangibleness means we rarely stop to reflect about its importance, its key role in our lives, and how critical it is for our physical and emotional balance.

In the next few chapters, we will get to know the ways in which the brain processes music, its many therapeutic uses in the 21st century and the ways we can consciously incorporate it in our everyday life, in order to achieve a healthy and balanced life.

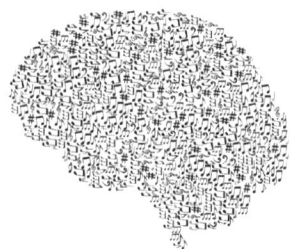

Chapter 2

MUSIC AND COGNITION

We have all experienced the excitement of listening to a song that reminds us of a special moment in our lives, a certain period, a love, a separation. We know intuitively that when we listen to music our brain is taking part in a much more complex process than just listening to and processing a sound.

Numerous cultural traditions around the world recognize that sound isn't just auditory perception. For example, the Tuvan people, throat singers from the south of Siberia,[38] paint landscapes through sound and vocal gestures, and the Yoreme community in Mexico paint sonic drawings to transform their spatial perception through specific musical progressions.[40]

From a neurological standpoint, many studies have shown evidence that sound affects the frontotemporal parietal regions of the brain, which causes a multimodal processing of sound.[41] This means that when we hear a sound, our brain activates a number of processes all at once, which connect various regions of the brain. These connections make it possible, for example, for Alzheimers' patients, who have lost the ability to recognise even their closest relatives, to recognise or perform complex melodies.[42] They also make it possible for a song to make us dance or for us to decipher complex poetic metaphors in the lyrics.

In fact, our perception of the world depends on our ability to establish multimodal cross-connections within our senses.[43]

To understand these processes, many researchers have studied synesthesia, a condition which allows some people to perceive sensory stimuli using two or more senses at once. Coming from the Greek words "syn", which means "with", and "aisthesis", which means sense, synesthesia occurs in approximately 1 out of every 200 people in the United States,[44] with these people possessing a neurobiological hyperconnectivity that allows them to involuntarily perceive simultaneous stimuli, e.g. see the colors of sounds or listen to tastes etc.[45]

A famous example of a synesthetic person throughout history is the Russian composer, Alexander Scriabin (1872-1915), who could see the colours of music and suggested the creation of an *Omni-art*, a synthesis of music, philosophy and religion with an aesthetic language that unified music, image, sound, drama, poetry and dance. With this, he aimed to bring the human mind towards a higher and more complex reality, towards ecstasy. His interest in the relationship between sound and colour led him to compose *Le poème de l'extase* and *Prométhée, Le poème du feu, op.60*, works which mixed both these elements. He was so convinced that the experience of colour would intensify the auditory experience that he declared that the audience would absorb his *Prométhée* more completely if they bathed in the colour which corresponded to the music.[46]

Although only a small percentage of the global population is synesthetic, in 1929, with his famous experiment *Kiki, Boulba*, Köhler showed that 90% of participants related the word *Kiki* to an angular shape and the word *Boulba* to a rounded shape.[47]

Perhaps you yourself relate sharp sounds to the cold or to sour tastes, or deep sounds to dark, warm and rounded colours. Everyone has different associations with music, colour, textures and tastes, which shows that a significant amount of the general population exhibits synesthetic tendencies and therefore, multimodal perception exists, although it is not present in such an extreme form, as it is in those with synesthesia. This hypothesis is used to study the different levels of connectivity in the brain upon hearing a sound and therefore it argues in favour of the relationship between music, movement and emotion.[48]

How do we hear?

Understanding how we hear is the first step in understanding the perception of sound. A sound is essentially the impression made in the ear by a mix of vibrations that are spread by an elastic medium, such as air or water. The sound is spread from one particle to the next. When the sound reaches the ear, for example a word or a song, it is initially captured by our auditory system in a basic or elemental form. The human ear can capture sounds between 20 Hz - 20 kHz. It is most sensitive between 2 kHz and 5 kHz. It has been noted that the upper limit decreases with age.

The auditory system is marvellous because it is capable of detecting even the most minute variations in pressure. The ear is divided into the outer, middle and inner ear. Soundwaves travel from the outer ear, through the ear canal, making the eardrum vibrate. In turn, this makes the three ossicles in the middle ear, known as the hammer, anvil and stirrup, move. These vibrations travel through the oval window to the fluid in the cochlea of the inner ear, stimulating thousands of little cilia cells. These vibrations turn into electric impulses which the brain perceives as sound. If any one of these components loses its ability to move, whether this be the result of an infection, a scar or a pathology, it will have a negative effect on the auditory capacity. Despite being a very sensitive organ, luckily the ear has mechanisms to protect itself against very intenses sound, or sounds with a very high frequency.

The perception of sound, however, is much more complex that the mere transmission of waves though an auditory apparatus - this is just the beginning of a complex process.

Upon listening to music, numerous regions in the brain are activated, in what we call multimodal perception, in other words, a multitude of processes, areas and networks are activated, which means we are not just limited to listening to the sound. The perception of sound is linked to emotion, memory, images. Studying the perception of sound and of music implies studying the mechanisms of cerebral cognition.

What is cognition and how is it studied?

Cognition is a human characteristic without which we could not survive. It has been defined in many ways, from the processes of general thinking and the intellectual capacity that includes memory, attention and learning, right until the acquisition of knowledge of surroundings and sensory systems. It also includes the processing and acquisition of languages.

Although there is an overlap of the regions of the brain which are involved in carrying out the different cognitive functions, there is also a certain specificity depending on which cognitive abilities we are referring to.

The part of the brain which is usually associated with complex cognitive processes such as episodic memory, reasoning and spatial abilities[49] is the prefrontal cortex.[50]

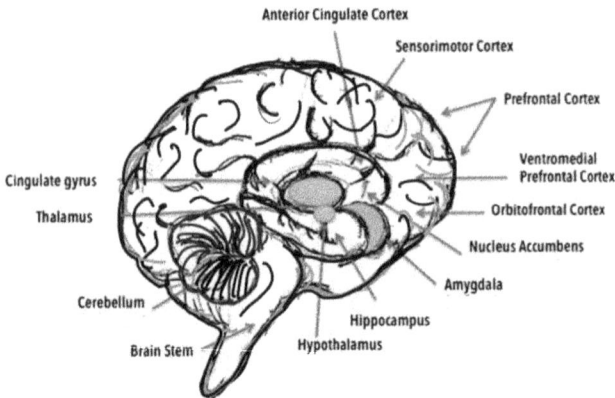

Anterior Cingulate Cortex
Sensorimotor Cortex
Prefrontal Cortex
Ventromedial Prefrontal Cortex
Orbitofrontal Cortex
Nucleus Accumbens
Amygdala
Hippocampus
Hypothalamus
Brain Stem
Cerebellum
Thalamus
Cingulate gyrus

Meanwhile, the control of attention can be attributed to the convolution of the anterior cingulate cortex inside the frontal lobe,[51] although, as it is also necessary to carry out other cognitive functions in an effective manner, it is located in multiple regions of the brain.[52] Attention can be defined in many ways, as it implies a system of functions which includes the ability to focus on a task and at the same time, filter out the unnecessary stimuli for the task at hand. It simultaneously involves different regions of the brain,[53] as it links various cognitive and perceptive processes and motor actions.[54,55]

Memory can be linked to the prefrontal and temporal regions of the brain, in particular to the hippocampus.[56] These processes are carried out by the limbic system, which is also responsible for the processes of learning alongside the thalamus and the cerebellum, and memory, a structure associated with the learning of complex movements necessary for playing musical instruments.[57]

The cognitive processes which involve attention, memory and learning are only possible due to the stimuli acquired by the senses, through our system of perception, that includes touch, taste, sight and sound, in fact so much so that often cognition is defined as the learning that we develop thanks to information obtained from our surroundings through the senses.

Until relatively recently, studies about cognition were dominated by two paradigms, the cognitivist and the adaptationist. These models aim to explain how exactly the brain works, how mental operations are carried out, and what evolutionary mechanisms have contributed to the development of these cerebral abilities. These ways of understanding and studying the brain have influenced the way in which we study the perception and cognition of music.

We have to go back to the 1940s to find the beginnings of the cognitive science we now understand. In the boom of the cybernetic movement, researchers of the brain introduced the idea that mental processes resembled the functioning of computers.[58] The influence of this model on the study of cognition promoted a disembodied view of cognition and of musical experience. Under this paradigm, cognition of music was studied just as an analysis of symbols, concepts, representations, ignoring the role of emotions and corporal perception.

In contrast, the cognitivist conception of the mind promotes a view that the mind is organised into modules which gradually adapt to the extent that they evolve.[59] As a result, the complexity of human thinking is analysed in terms of evolution of modules of cognition that adapt through natural selection in order to aid the survival of the individual.[60]

Numerous authors have questioned the cognitivist-adaptionist model, believing that it does not take epigenetic or environmental factors into account, in other words, it partially ignores the influence of surroundings and by doing so, it creates a division between mind, body and environment. [61]

In recent times, a paradigm has been developed which understands cognition as a permanent process of exchange and conversation between the body and the surroundings, in which multimodal perception, sensory-motor activity, emotions and metabolic processes are in constant and continuous movement.[62,63]

Studying the perception and processing of music is of great interest to neuroscientists as it requires the simultaneous activation of multiple parts of the brain. For example, when we learn to play a musical instrument, we are simultaneously carrying out multiple motor and sensory actions, which are very demanding at a cognitive level.[64,65]

Let's imagine a piano or guitar student, who presses the keys or the strings and at the same time is reading the score. In this action which seems so simple, the brain perceives through seeing the notes on the score and translates them into movements. The brain simultaneously captures the sounds produced and corrects the movements.

The act of playing an instrument requires extremely specific functions that are spread around numerous regions of the brain. The more complex the music, the more attention it requires. The musical experience also includes even more elements like rhythm, tempo and tuning. However, when we talk about cognition of music, we're not only referring to processes which happen when you perform an instrument, as even listening to music, without playing it, also stimulates various zones of the brain and requires complex processes. Our relationship with music could be both active and passive.

Without a doubt, the musical experience is much more than the mere acquisition and processing of auditory stimuli. We perceive music and we give it meaning according to the social, cultural and historical context in which we live. The meaning of music for us depends on our context, but at the same time, music gives meaning to this context. In other words, music should not be thought of as something external, separate from us. To exist, it has to be an integral part of our psychological, historical and social environment. This inspired Small to argue that music should not be used as a noun, but rather as a verb, and he proposed the term musicking.

"Musicking is participating, in whatever capacity, in a musical performance, whether you are performing, listening. learning or practising, providing material for the performance (what we call composing) or dancing. Sometimes, we can even extend its meaning to include the person who checks tickets at the door or the people who move pianos and drum kits, or those who set up instruments or do soundchecks or clean up after everyone has left. All of these people are also contributing to the nature of this event which is a musical performance".[66]

Looking at it this way, music does not rely on objects external to us, music is not defined as the instruments or objects that make it, it is not defined as the people that play it. In reality, music is an action, something that we do, something we participate in, whether that be through listening, performing, dancing, practicing, etc.[67] *Musicking* is an action which is carried out, lived, experienced by the body - a body which is in a permanent relationship and conversation with its surroundings.

This view of music takes us away from the cognitivist model which reduces music to a concept, symbol or mental process and brings us closer to a model that needs the body; music is lived through the body, it is embodied. By doing so, it is placed into the social, historical and cultural environment. In other words, when we *musick*, we do it from a social, historical place, from a gender, an age, a culture, a level of education. We can only musick from a body in constant conversation with its surroundings, in constant change and biological adaptation. The body becomes a space for cultural expression, shaped by our environment and culture.

Perhaps it would surprise you to know that in many cultures, the concept of music doesn't exist, at least not in the way we know it to be in the West, a purely sonorous experience. In many places, what we call music is an integral and inseparable part of cultural practices that include dance, performing arts and even paintings. For example, the Patua people in East Bengal in India, a nomad caste of painters of scrolls, sing through the scenes that they paint, that is to say, painting and music are inseparable. In many other cultures, music and dance are the same thing, which makes sense as they both involve movement. When the movement of the body produces sound, it produces music and when this movement is expressed purely as a form, it is dance.

If you think about it, when we are making music, we are always moving, not just to produce sound, for example when we move our fingers to play an instrument, but rather we also carry the rhythm in our bodies, we dance. Can you imagine a salsa, bossanova, opera or rock singer performing without moving? Or a jazz performer playing their instrument stood frozen like a statue? It is impossible to imagine this because music implicitly implies movement.

It is then easy to understand that the perception of music is much more complex than the processing of a sound in a concrete area of the brain; far from it, the sound is the initial stimulus that births a number of processes in multiple areas of the brain. Upon receiving the musical stimulus, many types of connections begin, which impact spheres such as emotion, motor functions, memory, affection and an endless number of metabolic reactions that take place in the body.

The study of music confirms that there is no such thing as division of body and mind, nor does thinking exist as an abstract thing, a mere processing of symbols at a neuronal level. Cognition begins in the body, a body which cannot be separated from the environment which provides it stimuli.

According to this view, cognitive processes are not limited only to the brain, but rather pass through the body without limiting it. Everything in my surrounding environment which I touch, see, listen to, the objects and devices I use all form part of my cognition, a cognition extended and embedded in the environment.

This ecological view of cognition is what we call 4E cognition. It is called *4E* because it refers to the four concepts which begin with the letter E: *Embodied, Extended,*[69] *Enacted* and *Embedded.*[70]

The evolution of the study of cognition of music, which in a relatively short time has transformed from the cognitivist-adaptavist model to a multimodal 4E cross-model, reflects the trend of Western society in the 21st century to question the compartmentalization of knowledge, to accept the need of transdisciplinarity and to recognise that we are inseparable from the environment that surrounds us.

Now that we understand how we perceive and process sounds, we will discover how the marvelous brains of musicians work.

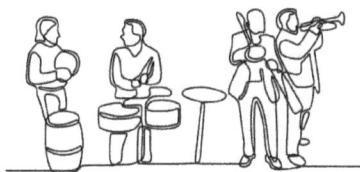

Chapter 3

THE MARVELOUS
BRAIN OF
MUSICIANS

The brain is a marvelous and often mysterious organ. We still have a lot to discover about how it works, about the thousands of processes that are constantly happening even during the most simple of tasks.

In complex activities, like playing an instrument or singing, our brain activates multiple zones and functions at the same time. It simultaneously activates cortical mechanisms related to the execution of highly specific cognitive and motor functions and multiple sensory systems. To put it simply, playing music is actually the brain carrying out a high-performance task.

In fact, many studies which compare the cognitive skills of musicians with those of non-musicians of the same age show that the former performs functions significantly better and responds more quickly in all cognitive skills tests, showing that musical training is a protective factor against neuro-cognitive aging. While playing an instrument, we are exercising our perception, attention, memory and learning processes.[71]

Knowing these benefits should inspire us to include music in our daily activities, especially if we think about how we live in a society where life expectancy is increasing day by day, meaning it is likely we will live for quite a long time, hopefully with full access to our cognitive skills. This awareness is very important if we consider that one in every nine people over the age of 65 and one in three over the age of 85 have cognitive limitations.[72] These figures tend to multiply when we take into account that between 2019 and 2100, the percentage of people over 80 years in the European Union is expected to multiply by 2.5%, a jump from 5.8% to 14.6%. In the US, it is predicted that by 2060, the population of elders is expected to increase by 105.2%.

How do we get to such an age while still maintaining our cognitive skills? What can we do so that the natural decline in our cognitive abilities is slow and we reach old age while still in possession of our mental faculties?

There are many factors which determine cognitive aging, including level of education, physical activity and diet.[73] In other words, once again we can see that our daily habits are the most important factor to maintain our mental and physical health. For example, a lot of evidence has shown that habits, such as reading or playing an instrument reduce the risk of developing dementia.[74] What these protective activities have in common is that all of them present a cognitive challenge - they are activities which require the simultaneous coordination of various functions.

What could be a bigger challenge than playing an instrument and singing at the same time? Or learning different pieces which require the development of increasingly complex technical skills? When we play an instrument a number of sensory systems (sound, sight, touch) need to be coordinated with our motor activity,[75] and this coordination also requires us to keep constantly changing the focus of attention. The development of these skills is the reason why professional musicians get higher marks in all cognitive tests compared to non-musicians.[76] It has also been shown that musicians in professional orchestras, who require a higher level of cognitive complexity in their activities, develop dementia less frequently than the general population.[77]

Without a doubt, musical practice is a protective factor for the brain.

But are there differences between the brain of a musician and that of a non-musician?

There is a lot of evidence that musical experience shapes the brain structurally[78] and physiologically.[79] From a structural viewpoint, in other words, the makeup of the brain and its different regions, we know that the anterior part of the corpus callosum of musicians is larger than that of non-musicians. This is also the case with the central sulcus in both hemispheres of the brain, which is deeper for musicians, and with the parts of the brain associated with the primary auditory cortex, Broca's area and the inferior frontal gyrus.[80] The cerebellum of musicians is also larger. Some studies have shown that people who play instruments have more grey material in the primary and somatosensory motor, premotor, frontal parietal and inferior frontal gyrus areas.[81]

However, the most remarkable differences between the brain of musicians and non-musicians are not structural, rather those related to perception and processing of sounds and their different features. Musicians process multisensory musical stimuli more quickly[82] and develop greater skills like auditory memory, attention and the ability to distinguish keys.[83]

Comparing the results of musicians and non-musicians in variations of rhythm and key shows that the former are quicker than the latter, which isn't surprising due to musical training. What is surprising, however, is that non-musicians detect differences more easily with the left ear, while musicians don't show any preference, which is also called lateralization.

This difference could boil down to the fact that musical training stimulates inter-hemispheric communication[84] which results in a level of cortical reorganisation more pronounced in those who begin to study music at a young age, as the brain is more malleable in the first few years of development.[85] This means that for musicians, the two hemispheres of the brain share functions and communicate with each other more fluidly.

Just a few years of musical training during infancy (a minimum of two years according to some studies) can have an impact on the neuronal codification in adulthood, even years after not studying.[86] These positive effects can extend to the sphere of memory, attention and cognitive skills in general. The good news is that even if we haven't received musical training during our childhood, simply growing up in an environment full of auditory stimuli leads to cerebral plasticity.[87] Even better news is knowing that this cerebral plasticity will remain throughout our whole life, in other words, at whatever age, we can reap in the benefits of music.

Musical practice doesn't just strengthen useful skills for the performance of music, like for example being able to identify the sound of an instrument in an ensemble, but rather it also leads to a more precise and efficient processing of sound, important for other types of communication.[88] This ability to extract meaning from complex sonic landscapes is an important factor in the transferring of skills to non-musical domains, such as the learning of languages. For example, musicians are more able to pick up languages or identify errors in second languages.[89]

Whether it be distinguishing a sound, or recognizing a voice in a noisy place, the brain of a musician is able to discern an auditory signal and extract it from a complex sonic landscape more easily than the brain of a non-musician.

Although I have not explicitly mentioned it, what we are talking about when highlighting the plasticity of the brain is our habits and the impact that they have on our health or sickness. When we consider that only two years of musical training during childhood can heighten cognitive abilities, we are recognising the importance of maintaining habits that stimulate our brain, and our body in all its aspects, in other words, placing myself in an environment rich in cognitive stimuli, whether they are sonic, visual, interpersonal, etc, is imperative for my cognitive health. Throughout life, we continuously redesign our neural routes. By being exposed to sonic stimuli, our auditory system dynamically modulates the processing of signals which have been accumulated through time, developing a sensory experience. In other words, all my auditory experiences fuse together so that my brain learns cognitive and sensory processes through experience, and my responses to stimuli slowly form. Sounds which we have picked up on in the past help shape our automatic response to new sounds in the present.

Through this experience, we learn to select the auditory stimuli most relevant to us. With time, this accumulated experience births a *"neuronal signature"* of experience, which is different for each person[90] This neuronal signature causes, for example, a musician's brain to respond and adjust to the specific timbre of the instrument they play. In other words, the brain responds better to this familiar timbre than to the sound of another instrument. The wider the stimuli we receive, the wider too becomes our spectrum of pleasure, in other words, we learn to enjoy new sounds.

The existence of this "neuronal signature" explains

why, for example, the style of musical performance also affects the processing of sound. This can be clearly seen in jazz musicians who show a greater sensitivity to subtle acoustic variations in their cerebral responses if you compare them with musicians from other genres, as they are used to improvisation and are hyper aware of changes in the music to which they have to adapt in a matter of seconds.[91]

During a musical performance, there are also multiple physiological changes, such as hormones and neurotransmitters being released, which are chemical substances that send, receive, amplify or modulate messages in the brain and in the whole body.[92] This chemical *cocktail* is responsible, among other things, for the phenomenon commonly known as "performance adrenaline", the anxiety we feel before going on stage that sometimes becomes the dreaded stage fright.

You don't have to be a musician to have experienced this anxiety, for example think of when you might have had to do a presentation in public or go out on stage. This anxiety we feel just before going on stage, that mix of desire to finally get out on stage and share the work we have dedicated so much time to, the fear of thinking that it won't turn out as we hope and the apprehension of how the public will react sometimes paralyses us. Your heart starts beating fast, your breathing gets shaky, your hands become sweaty and cold, your senses are heightened and you become more sensitive.

For some people, this anxiety paralyzes them, turning into that infamous stage fright, while others overcome it and rush out on stage to perform their music.

All of these feelings are due to the release of many substances including endorphins, neurotransmitters known as natural opiates, as they produce a similar effect to morphine. These endorphins reduce breathing rate and produce a vasodilating effect which lowers blood pressure, and are produced normally in situations of stress, helping to control pain, body temperature, sexual activity, memory, hunger and thirst. Its most notable effects are the slowing of breathing rate and decrease in blood pressure, due to its vasodilating effect.[93]

During a singer's performance, for example, they are essential to regulate breathing, the foundation for the production of sound.

During a performance, there is also a release of serotonin, a neurotransmitter which has a large effect on behavior, mood, memory and attention.[94] For the performer, it is especially important as it helps to recognize the emotional states in the facial expressions of those who are surrounding them, and it improves attention and memory, and leads to the best possible performance.[95]

Another part of this neurotransmitter *cocktail*, which heightens our senses during musical performance is dopamine, which is involved in both thinking as well as regulation of motor functions and mood. Dopamine is released in situations of environmental change, and it helps us adapt and it prepares us physically and emotionally for what is to come. Dopamine is linked to the prediction of rewarding events, which is speculated to be the origin of aesthetic criticism.[96]

However, the neurotransmitter which is more often linked to musical performance is adrenaline, a substance which incidentally acts like a hormone and like a neurotransmitter on multiple levels. Adrenaline is released in stressful "fight or flight" situations. Primordial mechanisms are activated, the same mechanisms which were activated in the first hominids in their fight for survival against the elements, and these mechanisms directly tie us to our remote ancestors. In these situations, the body increases its heart rate and undergoes vasoconstriction in order to send blood to the skeletal muscles to prepare us to defend ourselves from danger. Our energy and strength are increased and our breathing rate, blood pressure and blood sugar level elevates. Adrenaline prepares us for battle, but its effects can be devastating during a musical performance, especially during a singing performance, where we need a regulated breathing rate, and so to speak, we need to take it down an octave to be in complete awareness and control.

An important part of musical training, especially for singers, whose instrument is our own body, is learning to observe ourselves and be aware of our body in order to balance the chemical storm inside us during a public performance. This is why singers study relaxation, breathing and body awareness techniques, so that we can be fully conscious and in control during our performance. The goal of these exercises is to reach our full potential, to give 110% when we're out on stage.

Although musicians, like elite athletes, use these exercises to achieve their peak performance, learning these techniques has a positive impact on their general health. Musical practice and performance present a number of unique challenges for the nervous system that cause the brain of musicians to be different to that of non-musicians, and cause them to develop cognitive skills which protect them from the degeneration associated with aging.

These findings should be enough to encourage us to

play an instrument or sing, not just for the positive changes to the brain but also because it has been proved that musical practice makes us happier, and improves our quality of life.

Music helps us socialize, connect to one another, express ourselves, share with the world who we are or what we want to be. When we sing, play an instrument, attend a concert or dance, we express ourselves in the most authentic way, we introduce ourselves to others as who we truly are, with no filter. We free our bodies and vibrate together with others and with the universe, expressing the purest essence of who we are and by doing this, we merge with a group, forming part of something bigger, a community.

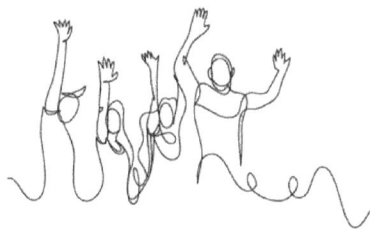

Chapter 4

PLEASURE, EMOTION AND MUSIC

I remember when I was ten years old, when I started to sing, often people who listened to me would tell me that they got goosebumps, and at the time I didn't understand exactly what they meant by that, although I felt as though it was something positive since they said it like praise. With time, I myself began to feel different sensations while listening to music which I liked a lot; the pit in my stomach, the knot in my throat, goosebumps and even the desire to cry.

Later on, I learnt that more than 50% of the population experience these types of physiological and emotional reactions while they listen to music or live through similar intense aesthetic experiences. Music has the power to alter our physical and emotional state, which is perhaps why music is all around us these days, it accompanies us in all the circumstances and moments of our life. In fact, many studies have shown that one of the most important reasons to listen to music throughout the day is to experience and regulate emotional states.[97] Some of these experiences can be so intense that they can trigger long-term effects on the person's wellbeing.[98]

The emotions caused by music are intimately linked to memory, they trigger our past experiences and they make it easier to access autobiographical memory. This explains why we link certain songs to certain moments in our lives that are important or packed full of emotions. Loss, pain, love, heartbreak are all associated with songs, which become the soundtrack of a certain period of our lives, referential moments in our existence, like sound chapters of our autobiographies.

The ability to identify emotions in music appears at an early age during development. As early as some time between the second and fourth month of life, we are able to relate pleasant feelings with consonant sounds and unpleasant feelings with dissonant sounds.[99] Around the third and fourth year, we gain the ability to identify happy music and around the sixth, we recognise a wide range of emotions in music, including sadness, fear and anger.[100]

Initially, we form connections with basic musical emotions, such as associating fast-paced music with joy and slow-paced music with sadness. As time goes on, we gradually refine our ability, being able to link different emotional states with more complex characteristics of music; for example, we associate sadness with music in a minor key and happiness with music in a major key.

This raises a number of questions: what do we mean when we talk about emotion? What goes on inside our body when we listen to music? How are music, pleasure and emotion connected?

Defining emotions is complicated. From the dawn of time, man has tried to explain them from different viewpoints, such as philosophy, psychology, and more recently neuroscience. According to the first philosophers, emotions were a category of feelings, separate from other proprioceptive or sensory sensations. From the 19th century, with the rise of experimental psychology, a number of theories emerged making it difficult to reach a consensus about what an emotion is made up of.[101]

Some emotions seem automatic, consistent and universal[102], and others seem to be determined by the sociocultural context in which they are triggered.[103] To make things even more difficult, many scientists discuss whether emotional experiences are a result of autonomous physiological changes[104] or whether they are triggered by environmental changes,[105] - it seems like the age old question of whether the chicken or the egg came first. The distinction between basic and complex emotions[106] gets lost in these discussions, making it even more elusive to define.

One of the most widespread theories, initially hypothesised by Darwin,[106] proposes that there are basic, uncompromising emotions, which come as a result of evolution[108] and respond to adaptative, universal, biologically determined processes.[109] A prime example of this is fear, a behavioural motivator in response to a threat, that seems to have a common psycho-physiological response[110] and seemingly is processed mainly in a part of the brain called the amygdala.[111] However, the amygdala is related to many other processes, including the recognition of emotions in the music,[112] which confirms that there aren't localized regions of the brain for specific emotions.

One of the main criticisms of this theory is that there is no consensus about what the basic emotions[113] are and how many of them exist. Some researchers have stated that the only basic emotions are pleasure and fear, however the most widely accepted definition includes basic emotions such as joy, wrath, fear, sadness, disgust, embarrassment, surprise, scorn, interest, blame, acceptance and anticipation.[114]

In contrast, the theory of assessing emotions focuses on how we judge, evaluate and understand stimuli, in other words, more than the stimuli itself which triggers the emotion,[115] it is important how we assess it, and this depends on cultural and environmental factors. This explains how a single stimulus can cause different emotional reactions in different people.[116]

Finally we come to the constructionist approach to emotion, which focuses on the effects of stimuli on the cultural, social and biological surroundings. In other words, according to this paradigm, emotional response and it's varying intensity are the result of the interaction between the stimulus, the culture, the society and somatic markers, similar to the 4E model of cognition mentioned earlier. In this context, emotions and social interactions make up an unbreakable system, in other words, emotions are expressed socially and historically and are recognised, simulated and controlled in different ways, in accordance with the social, historical, class and gender context.

Therefore, when we try to understand the emotional effects of music, we must keep in mind its cognitive, social, therapeutic and aesthetic effects on the listener.

In 1871, Darwin stated: "Music awakens various emotions within us, but not the most awful ones like horror, fear, anger etc. It awakens the gentler emotions, like tenderness and love, that quickly turn into devotion."[117] These statements of Darwin have recently been confirmed by researchers that found that although music is able to produce a wide range of emotions, it usually stimulates positive emotional states, like happiness-euphoria and nostalgia-longing.[118] Emotions like wrath, irritation, boredom-indifference or anxiety-fear are found more often in daily emotions rather than when we listen to music. Zentner, Grandjean and Scherer also showed that music usually triggers positive reactions like relaxation and joy than negative ones like aggression, anxiety, depression and wrath.[119]

Darwin also stated that emotions generated by music fulfil an evolutionary role, that, along with songs, dances or rites of a community, foster social ties, leading to survival. An example of this are the sounds that a baby and its carer exchange. The musical properties of this first communication have been shown to be essential for the survival of the infant.

Recent authors have suggested that there are two types of emotions, the utilitarian ones, linked to the interest and wellbeing of an individual, and musical aesthetics. According to researchers, the terms used by subjects to describe emotions that they feel while listening to music correspond with the nine musical aesthetic emotions: amazement, transcendence, tenderness, nostalgia, peace, power, joy, tension and sadness.[120]

A controversial point that arises from this analysis is whether music evokes emotions in listeners or whether they just recognize the emotion expressed by the musical piece. In the first instance, musical stimulus triggers a series of psychological, physiological or motor reactions, like for example, the feeling of calmness, relaxation or happiness, or the tendency of our bodies to follow the rhythm. A different situation from this would be when we recognize that a piece is sad or happy, but this doesn't trigger emotional responses, in other words, my relationship with the music is purely cognitive. I recognize that the music is happy but I don't feel happy or I listen to sad music but feel happy, that is to say, the perceived emotions do not coincide with the emotions felt.

In general, scientific literature suggests that the amygdala and numerous regions of the temporal lobe are the areas involved in the perception of emotion in music.

The ability to perceive music and the ability to perceive emotions in music have been clinically differentiated, having observed that patients with damage to their temporal lobes are impeded from recognizing emotions in music despite being perfectly able to perceive it.[121]

We also know that environmental and social factors determine our emotional response to music; it is not the same to listen to a sad song after a breakup or at a funeral of a loved one than listening to it as background music while I do other things or as Muzak in a lift.

Certain songs which are played in battlefields, in political or religious demonstrations, or in football stadiums have the effect of energizing, uniting and exciting a group of people who share ideals and ideologies. This proves that emotions triggered by music are also linked to non-musical factors. The same song can trigger different physiological and emotional responses in different contexts.[122]

A way to evaluate the emotional response to music is through analyzing psycho-physiological responses to it. The most common responses include changes in blood pressure, pulse, skin conductance and changes in muscle tension. It has also been shown that upon listening to clips of musical pieces which express sadness, fear, anxiety, the level of physiological excitement of the body changes. Sad music alters, above all, heart rate, blood pressure, skin conductance and body temperature of listeners. Music which expresses fear causes, above all, changes the beats per minute of the pulse. Finally, happy music causes changes in breathing.

Within these observed changes, we can also find the so-called "goosebumps" or "the chills", which I mentioned at the start. This feeling, described as pleasurable, consists of a type of electricity that begins in the neck and is felt the whole way down the spine, is usually associated with making your hair stand on end.

Defining pleasure is also complicated. We surely all agree that pleasure is subjective, relative, and that what is pleasurable for you is revolting for others. Human beings are as simple or as complex as our pleasures.

Several authors differentiate between the so-called fundamental pleasures, the necessary ones for survival of the species, like sex, food, belonging to a group and those of "high priority", more conscious pleasures, such as financial earnings, social acceptance, religious beliefs, musical and aesthetic pleasure. Although these pleasures are not necessary for survival, they activate the same parts of the brain as fundamental pleasures.[123]

Despite the brain having many networks and circuits related to the reward system, it seems as though pleasure mechanisms are much more specific, and in other words, rarer. Some of these structures that play a role in pleasure are tethered to the back of the brain, for example in the striatum or in the brain stem and some are found in the cerebral cortex,

It also seems that there are very small regions in the subcortex structures, called *"hedonic hotspots"* by researchers, which are separated but also connected like an archipelago and are involved in pleasure responses.[124]

Barridge and Kringelbach described the cycle of pleasure, which starts with an initial desire, an anticipation that, at a cerebral level, triggers the release of dopamine. When we obtain and enjoy the object of desire, for example experiencing an orgasm or winning a bet, other neurotransmitters called opiates are activated. After having escaped the initial tension, we enter into a phase of learning and relaxation. These phases of pleasure combine conscious and unconscious elements, in other words, we can consciously identify some of these states, but there are factors which do not enter our consciousness and operate at a much deeper level.

The same pleasure cycle also happens with the musical experience. Neuroimage studies of subjects that experience goosebumps when listening to music show activation of the bilateral amygdala, the left hippocampus, the ventromedial prefrontal cortex, and various other regions related to pleasure and euphoria.[125] Also the ventral striatum is activated, a region associated with the processing of gratification, hedonistic impact, learning and motivation.[126]

Neuroimaging scans such as PET and fMRI show evidence that listening to music which we like activates the same regions of the brain as those activated when we experience euphoria, when we receive erotic stimuli or when we eat chocolate. For this reason, many refer to the sensation of "goosebumps" caused by music as a musical orgasm.

Like always, there are people who experience musical pleasure more intensely. These differences are determined by a number of factors, including personality type and also genetic factors. This is what happens to those with congenital musical anhedonia[127] who don't experience any pleasure while listening to music. This condition affects 5.5% of the population,[128] though it can also be a result of neurological damage.

There is no doubt that music connects with emotion and produces pleasure, just think of how many times you have listened to a song, or performed in a concert, and felt a rush of emotions, or when you have felt energized at a fast-paced rhythm. As performers, we know that through music, we can express certain emotions that can't be communicated through words. The minute we begin our performance, it's as though time stops. When a musician has moved past the stage of technical learning, they experience transcendent moments in which they connect intimately with music, they become one with sound. In these moments, they reach an almost mystical state of absolute connection with the present, they truly live in the now and they freely express the musical message.

For singers, this moment represents the meeting point between music and poetry. Music and poetry merge with singing in a profoundly cathartic and transcendent way that links the modern-day singer with the ancestral figure of the shaman, the man/woman/medicine responsible for curing the community, for representing it, for floating between the real world and the world of ideas, of dreams.

During shamanic possession, the shaman, similar to the modern musician, experiences all the beings, all the lives and becomes one with the universe. As a singer, when I sing, I live a thousand lives, I experience every emotion, situation and event that although is not part of my reality, is close to me, as they are human experiences.

I always say that thanks to singing, I have been able to live as a man and a woman, a king and a beggar, an old person and a young person. I have been in love, abandoned, hopeful, alone, hurt and all-powerful.

While performing in full awareness of the poetry of the songs, I can express emotions which can only be accessed through the union of music and poetry. These moments of complete connection with the music, of mindfulness, that give us performers pleasure and happiness coincide with the moments that Csikszentmihalyi describes as *flow*. In these moments, every thought, intention, emotion and feeling is focused on the same goal.

When the flow experience takes place, we feel more connected, we reach a higher level of complexity, a complexity which is the result of two supposedly opposing movements: the differentiation which causes us to be authentic, unique, to separate ourselves from others, and the integration that brings us closer to others, that unites us, that joins us. The dialectic between these two supposedly contradictory forces produces a more complex and rich individual.

Whether it be performing or listening, music is a source of aesthetic pleasure. The great Russian composer, Igor Stravinsky described it like this:"

There is no better way to define the sensation produced by music than saying that it is the same feeling as the contemplation of the interaction of architectural forms.

Goethe understood it perfectly when he called architecture petrified music.

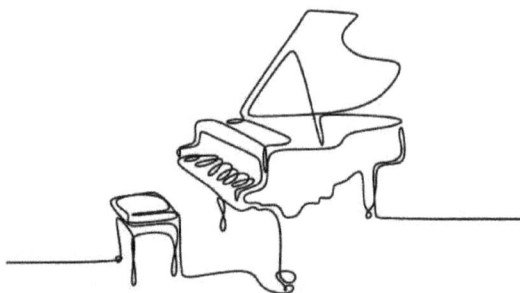

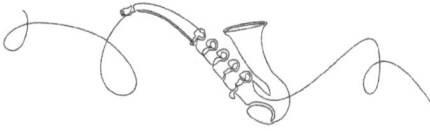

Chapter 5

MUSIC, HAPPINESS AND **THE MEANING OF LIFE**

From the dawn of time the search for happiness has been one of the deepest desires of humanity. A number of philosophies have equated a good life with a happy life. Many disciplines study this phenomenon, including psychology, philosophy, sociology and economics. It seems like everyone wants to be happy.

For some people, happiness seems to be a question of resources, of GDP. However, many studies have concluded that some of the most happy societies are not necessarily the richest. This idea challenges the values of the capitalist society where, in the last few decades, happiness has become a million dollar industry which leeches off our need to buy happiness. Every year, millions of self-help courses and books which suggest recipes and methods to achieve it are sold.

Mihaly Csikszentmihalyi, renowned researcher of happiness defined it as the ability to reach a state of flow:

> A state in which people are so involved in an activity that nothing else seems to matter; the experience is so enjoyable that people will continue to do it even at great cost, for the sheer sake of doing it.[129]

In his studies, he notes that all flow experiences share seven characteristics: they bring those who experience them a sense of competence in the activity, they combine action and concentration, they have clear objectives, they require complete and focused attention on the activity, they provide a sense of being in control, even if the situation itself isn't fully under control, they imply a loss of self-consciousness and of interpersonal connection and while experiencing them, all sense of time is lost.

There are two conditions which are always present in flow experiences. Firstly, participants feel that the activities seem like a challenge to their abilities and it provides them the opportunity to improve, to further develop their skills, and then, they should be able to evaluate their accomplishments so that they can define clear goals for the future. In these flow experiences, people develop their skills and continuously face more complex challenges, which keeps them motivated. Therefore these activities last for a long time, increasing the feeling of wellness.

Being a subjective state associated with the level of satisfaction that we have in different aspects of life, happiness is often confused with wellness, a concept which combines both the subjective aspects of happiness with objective aspects related to the quality of life. Wellness, a concept coined in the first decades of the 20th century, is defined as the optimum state of an individual, community or society as a whole. It is expressed in different ways in different cultural contexts, in fact, each society creates their own idea of wellness.

Bill Hettler, director of the National Wellness Institute in the United States[130] defined it as an active process through which people become conscious and choose options which bring them towards a fulfilled existence.[131] Hettler defined the six main dimensions of wellness, namely physical, social, emotional, intellectual, spiritual and occupational wellness.[132] Wellness is about achieving the balance of these six dimensions.

This holistic vision of the human being and his environment closely resembles a concept in medicine called homeostasis. At a biological level, homeostasis represents the optimum state in which organisms maintain a constant equilibrium and the physiological conditions to maintain life.

Personal homeostasis is therefore achieving this bio-psycho-social balance, which involves physical and psychological health and the ability to integrate and form an active part of a community. Illness occurs when there is a lack of balance in one of these dimensions. It makes sense that we link the concept of wellness to health, as wellness is a necessary condition to achieve health.

So what role does music play in happiness, wellness and consequently, in health? Recent studies carried out on professional musicians to evaluate their level of wellness at a mature and old age have shown that music is a key factor for maintaining their health and physical, cognitive and social skills during old age.[133]

Musical practice apart from providing intellectual and cognitive stimulation, also provides the feeling of belonging to a group and it facilitates the adaptation to changes associated with aging. Studies have shown that musicians stay healthy until very old, much older than the non-musical population, because playing an instrument requires them to maintain a healthy lifestyle, including their diet, posture, breathing, and it keeps them connected to their environment.

There is also a direct relationship between musical practice and happiness, as musicians constantly challenge themselves to learn new repertoires which leads them to this aforementioned flow. The feeling of happiness stems from the process of learning, achieving your goals, developing a sense of self-fulfillment, and feeling like you are achieving your potential. These findings are especially relevant in a society in which life expectancy has increased enormously in the last few years and hopefully will increase even further in years to come.

From a brain health point of view, many studies link listening and performing music to the increase of neurotransmitters which lead to relaxation, stimulate emotions such as enthusiasm, strengthen the immune system and facilitate social integration. The main neurotransmitters associated with these changes are dopamine, cortisol, serotonin and oxytocin.[134]

Although it was initially believed that oxytocin was only released during physical contact, such as the trust that develops between parents and children due to close contact, it has now been shown that group activities related to music, like singing in a choir, cause an increase in its levels, which explains how singing in a group can strengthen bonds of trust and cooperation between performers.[135]

Nuclear Magnetic Resonance (NMR) has also shown that upon receiving a musical stimulus, the cerebral arteries are oxygenated, triggering the release of neurotransmitters in many parts of the brain. Music is a catalyst in brain activity that promotes wellness, happiness and therefore a better quality of life.

One of the aspects that determine wellness is feeling like we have a purpose in life, an end goal, something that gives meaning and makes it worthwhile to be alive. This purpose or reason to live in Japanese is known as *Ikigai*, a concept that overlaps in many aspects with Csikszentmihalyi's definition of happiness, which relates the ability to experience states of flow with self-fulfillment and the feeling of being able to develop our skills to their maximum potential.

Music is marvelous because through it we can reach this state of flow in a collective or individual way. Our participation in this phenomenon of music gives rise to many ideas and actions, we respond to sensory impulses, we interpret and convey emotions.

Body, emotions and music fuse together, sound is embodied in the individual. While merging with sound, we become one with it and upon doing so, we experience one of the characteristics of flow; the merging of action and awareness.[136] This convergence of knowing and doing is especially meaningful in music, making it one of the activities that most easily produces this greatly desired state of happiness.

This statement itself should encourage *musicking*; it should encourage us to listen to more music throughout our lives, to study music from childhood, and to include it as an essential part of education.

Music acts as a tool for social integration, as a shared language that helps us to overcome our differences, to find similarities in our diversity, to build a consensus.

When we *musick*, we pour in every last drop of who we are, and our past, present and future, our memory, our perception of the now and our desire to share, to build all fuse together; everything merges when we musick.

To *musick* means to share an aesthetic experience in which I express my uniqueness and I give it generously to others. I hand it over so that they can experience it in their own way, so they can decode it and feel its presence in their body and their culture, in the values that define them, in their being. When I make music, I hand myself over, and by doing so, I leave a space for another to enter, for exchange, for growth, for transformation, for compassion.

This way of making music, of sharing the phenomenon of sound, is sadly far from the teachings of conservatories and institutions of professional musical education, where often intuition and playing by ear have been wiped out and the real use of music has been forgotten, in favour of a exceedingly rationalistic and technical learning.

Obviously a musician must learn technical skills which are developed through practice and through learning certain methodologies, but it is just as important to learn about the development of intuition, how to share music and incorporate it into all aspects of life, and also giving the same value to all musical traditions around the world.

In order to achieve a more healthy and happy, a more fair and compassionate society, music should be the base of the emotional, aesthetic and intellectual education for all the children of the world, as sagely demonstrated by the existence of the *Five Music Rights*, promulgated by the International Music Council.[137]

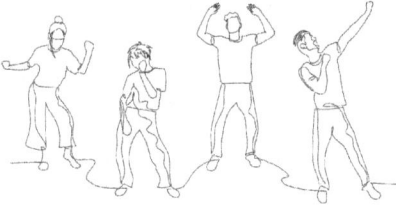

Chapter 6

RHYTHM, MOVEMENT AND HEALTH

"Everything flows, out and in; everything has its tides;
all things rise and fall; the pendulum-swing manifests in
everything; the measure of the swing to the right is the
measure of the swing to the left; rhythm compensates."

The Kybalion[138]

The universe is constantly expanding and moving in response to a rhythm and to a periodicity. Right from the smallest of subatomic particles to the biggest of stars, the universe is vibrating in a rhythmic movement. In the same way, our body is in constant movement, cells don't stop performing their biochemical processes, they regenerate.

Every new interaction with the environment causes changes within our brain and body. We are constantly changing right from birth to death.

Emilie Conrad Da'Oud stated that what we call a body is not material, but rather movement.[139] The body is a rhythmic orchestration of many forms of movement and sound, in which many different rhythms overlap; the rhythm of the heart, of breathing, of the digestive tract, the actions and reactions of the nervous system and even the cells and the auditory cortex that have their own inherent rhythm, independent of external stimuli.[140, 141]

When we are healthy, the rhythms of the body flow naturally. Physical or emotional illness are brought about by a change in the rhythm, they occur when we are off rhythm. Just like in a game of mirrors, we constantly reflect our internal, emotional, corporal movements in our social interactions and the environment around us. In the same way, the rhythms of our surrounding environment have a positive or negative impact on the rhythms of the body.

In Ancient Greece, philosophers like Plato proposed a difference between the knowledge gained through the body and that gained through reason, the latter which he linked to the soul, and which he placed more value to.

Following this Platonic tradition, Christianity condemned the knowledge gained through the body, associating it with sin and sexuality, placing the body on the opposite end of the spectrum to the desired virtues. Centuries later, Carthesian philosophers, with their famous "*I think, therefore I am*" further legitimised this way of thinking, giving rise to the philosophical dualism that influenced all the sciences and paradigms of thought, assigning greater value to the mind and to the rational than to the experiences acquired by the senses. This paradigm of thought, that remains even to this day a big part of academics, is completely the opposite of current neuroscientific evidence; just like we learnt in the chapter about music and cognition, the body is also a cognitive apparatus, through which we perceive the world and shape thought. There is no separation between body and mind, they are dependent on each other. Intelligence is first an intelligence of the body, an intelligence which develops by doing.

This means the experience we gain through our bodily interactions shapes our brains, creating new neural connections, a continuous process which happens throughout life thanks to our brain plasticity. Body, mind and environment make up an inseparable trinity. Health and illness are the result of the interaction between these three inseparable elements, we are bio-psycho-social beings.

Despite the evidence, and probably due to the fact that we've been living through centuries of this Carthesian paradigm, educational institutions, in all areas of knowledge - medicine, music, philosophy to name a few - keep perpetuating compartmentalized models of teaching which separate mind and body, assigning greater value to rational knowledge and separating science from the arts and humanities. As a result, medical training is mainly of a biological nature and arts, in particular, music is taught in a way that separates mind and body, turning musical performance into a purely rational, and therefore incomplete exercise.

Luckily, throughout history, in many cultures, forms of knowledge have recognized the importance of maintaining the balance between physical and emotional rhythms and the rhythms of our surrounding environment.

The first relationship we think of between rhythm and health is that which is usually found in shamanic ceremonies in which percussion instruments are played with a regularity and rhythms that induce altered states of consciousness, causing many diseases to be cured.

Now we know that the acoustic stimulation of drums affects the electrical activity of the brain and leads to synchronization or rhythmic entrainment. Entrainment is a physical phenomenon which causes the rhythms from different systems to synchronize. It was discovered in the 17th century by Christiaan Huygens, inventor of the pendulum of clocks, who observed in his workshop that the pendulums that were close to one another tended to synchronize.

There are different types of rhythmic entrainment: intra-individual entrainment, which happens when two or more systems within the individual themselves synchronizes, inter-individual which happens when two or more individuals synchronize, or inter-grupal, which happens when the activities of two or more groups synchronize.

We can observe this phenomenon, for example, when an energetic rhythm wakes up the autonomic nervous system, producing an increase in breathing, heart rate, cortisol, adrenaline and many other hormones, or when a musical stimulus affects heart rate, in other words, increases or decreases the number of times the heart beats per minute.

It is worth noting that Plato himself, in the *Timaeus*, one of his last works in which he describes numerous diseases, recommends to never move the soul without the body and the body without the soul, because it is the equilibrium of these two that keeps you in good health.

In the 11th century, the famous Arabic doctor Ibn Butlan recommended in the *Taqwim al-Sihha* - a text which had a great impact on Europe during the Middle Ages, known by its Latin translation *Tacuini or Theatrum sanitatis* - to make music and dance (*sonare et bailare*) as a way to maintain good health. The book, which lays the foundation for preventive medicine, outlines a set of recommendations to maintain good health which is the result of the balance of the so-called "six unnatural things" (*sex res non naturals*): (1) air, (2) food, (3) sleep, (4) movement and rest, (5) secretions and excretions, (6) emotions.

This codex, which in many ways remains current, is not just the source of information for doctors, but is also an exceptional iconographic source for the study of life during the Middle Ages. The remaining copies have been brightened with beautiful illustrations, which, in the section dedicated to *sonare et ballare*, show people dancing to the sound of music played by wind instruments. According to Ibn Butlan, the benefits of singing and dancing are received in equal parts by the performers and the audience.[142]

During the Middle Ages, there were records of a number of episodes which we would now call collective hysteria, when large groups of people started to dance frantically until the point of exhaustion.[143] Experts say these episodes, which some called Saint Vitus's dance, were a result of an epidemic of *Sydenham's chorea*, an infectious disease that produces involuntary muscle movements.

Throughout history, a good number of treated patients have described the benefits of movement and rhythm on their health, including the six books *De arte gimnastica* by Girolamo Mercuriale (1530-1606), published in 1569, the treaty *Sanitate tuenda* by Pierre Gontier, published in 1668 and the treaty by the French Michel Bicaise, published in 1669. According to Bicaise:"

> Music and sound make the mind dance by causing a harmonic motion, rhythm, swing. The swing of the body moves the mind.[144]

More than just discussing the benefits of movement, the treaties recommended specific dances for different diseases, depending on the age, gender, social class, profession and morphology of each patient. Different types of music were linked with the promotion of different virtues, for example, the Dorian mode, with its major key of today, was linked to virtues such as modesty, sobriety and prudence, while other modes and their related dances were linked to unbridled passions, which should be avoided.

In his book *Anatomy of melancholy*, published in 1621, Robert Burton links music, movement and emotion. In it, he recommends dance, hunting, walking and horse riding as a treatment for depression, which was then called melancholy and he explains how certain melodies and dance foster infatuation, which he calls the melancholy of love.

In the 19th century, the composer and teacher Emile Jacques-Dalcroze (1865-1950), the creator of the famous *eurhythmics* method stated that the rhythms of the body and of our surrounding environment, such as walking, running or the heartbeat, lead to the development of our intelligence right from infancy. According to Dalcroze, musical rhythm develops which we feel and we correlate our internal and external rhythms, in other ways, the rhythms of our own body and those of our surroundings.

Although Dalcroze's theories are relatively recent, the relationship between rhythm, movement and health dates back to more than 30,000 years ago, when shamanic ceremonies, considered the oldest systems of organised healing, were practised everywhere. In them, the shamans would play repetitive rhythms on the drums with regularity, which according to some studies was three taps a second, just the right number to evoke altered states of consciousness and trances in participants that would lead to healing.

The ancient practices of healing are linked to modern therapies such as the so-called *Neurodrumming*, a therapy which involves the use of drums and mantra chants following predetermined rhythms which have been shown to improve the cognitive and emotional capacities of participants, reducing levels of anxiety, stress and depression.

For people with autism and schizophrenia, there has been a lot of success when using a therapy known as *Rhythmic Entrainment Intervention* (REI), a treatment which consists of making a patient listen to the sound of drums to stimulate the central nervous system. This rhythm therapy has a positive effect at a cognitive level, an effect which is amplified when this activity takes place in a community setting.

Because of its benefits at a cognitive level, these types of therapy are considered mental or brain training, which most people traditionally associate with exercises to improve memory or maths problems, but in reality, this term can cover many areas, including participation in social activities which are essential for cognitive health.

Mental training is necessary and positive at every age as we know that neurogenesis, that is, the regeneration of brain cells, happens throughout your whole life.[145,146] Our brains are plastic, they regenerate constantly and they can be shaped and stimulated at any age.[147]

It has been shown that simple activities such as dancing,

or participating in a group drum activity,[148] can lead to longevity and the development of a healthy aging process as they require the activation of numerous cortical circuits and of complex cognitive processes. Attention, perception, mobility and many brain areas get exercised simultaneously. Although it seems easy to us, perceiving rhythm is both one of the most fundamental and one of the most complex experiences of our bodies.

What is rhythm?

Generally when we talk about a rhythmic song, we mean that the music induces a sense of temporary regularity, it is organized according to a pattern which gives it a regularity. However, there is a difference between the regularity of music, the rhythm of music and the rhythm that we perceive, in other words, when we talk about rhythm, we're talking about two phenomena, one external, the object sound with its regularity, and one internal, the subject which perceives the regularity of the sound.

The way in which we perceive rhythm is also influenced by the culture in which we are brought up. Many studies demonstrate that the perception of rhythm is different in Western and Eastern culture which confirms that biology and surroundings interact to shape our sense of rhythm.

Through dance, which is beautifully defined by some researchers as a type of organized energy that gives form to feeling,[150] the values of a society are represented. Dance becomes a space for resolving conflict and representing values that deeply express who we are as individuals and as a society.

In a study based on the analysis of Bolivian songs in Quechua, Stobart and Cross,[151] showed that when we listen to music, we perceive the beat in different ways depending on the culture in which we grow up. The authors attribute these differences to the rhythm of the Quechua languages, in other words, the "music" of the language we spoke, its prosody, determines how we perceive rhythm.

It has also been shown that the ability to perceive complex rhythms is increased when we have more exposure to different languages and types of music,[152] in other words, this skill can be developed if we stimulate our brain by exposing it to music and languages from different cultures.

Although all humans are born with the same skills to perceive simple and complex rhythms, they are then shaped by their culture. Already at nine months old, infants are able to distinguish different rhythms and show a preference for the rhythms of their own culture. When they reach twelve months, cultural preferences similar to those of adults arise, that is to say, a brief exposure to music develops our ability to perceive certain rhythms.[153]

Body movement and pleasure are related - it just takes us remembering moments in which we have danced to the rhythm of music for the body to start moving almost automatically, in sync with the music. Some studies have shown that we find music which is somewhat complex, but not too complex, pleasurable. To produce this pleasure, music should surprise us in some way, that is to say, it should have a structure that in any moment could suddenly change, whether it be removing a note or changing the rhythmic structure.[154]

Of course, what some find complex could be very simple for others, and therefore the pleasure that music produces depends fully on the person listening to it, on their cultural context. However, we could say that a certain level of syncope, that is, a certain level of irregularity and surprise in music makes it more pleasurable and more likely to make us move.

Although there is still a lot to discover about the brain mechanisms which produce pleasure and the ways in which rhythm and music affect us, we can state that pleasurable and playful activities like dancing and singing can greatly improve our quality of life. It has been shown that dancing or playing percussion instruments reduces anxiety, stress, as well as levels of testosterone and it regulates the hormone system.

Knowing the impact that our corporal experiences and habits have on our health grants us an incredible power, but also a great responsibility; we can shape our brain with our actions, slow down the aging process and live until an old age while maintaining good health. Let's dance!

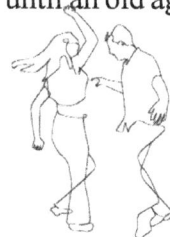

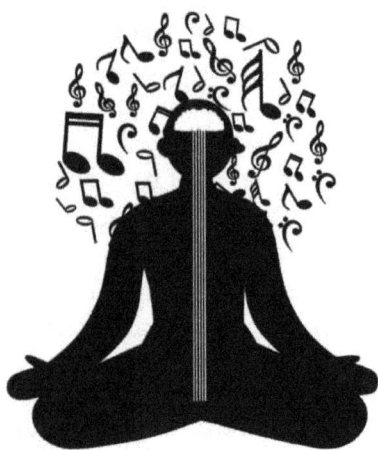

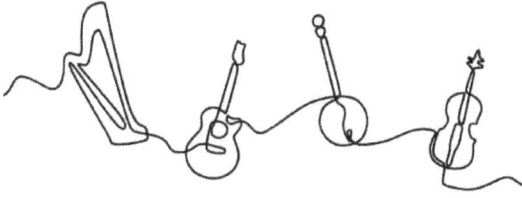

Chapter 7

MUSIC
IN PAIN
AND DEATH

Pain is a shared human experience, something which we have all experienced. Whether it's physical or emotional, pain is our body's way of warning us about an imbalance, something which is hurting us that we must pay attention to. According to the International Association for the Study of Pain (IASP), pain is a displeasurable subjective emotional or sensory experience related to tissue damage. By recognizing it is subjective, we accept that it cannot be generalized or compared between individuals, and we also understand that it is an experience which combines many physical, social, cultural and psychological elements. Pain is a complex and multidimensional phenomenon which should be dealt with in a transdisciplinary way.[155]

Our experience of pain is determined by factors as diverse as the memories we have of trips to the hospital, our anticipation before a specific procedure or our psychological state at the exact moment we're undergoing it.

Even more complex than physical pain, emotional pain can also not be measured, evaluated or compared, and the only thing we can say for certain is that we all suffer from it at some point during our lives and in these moments, music is there for us, it soothes us. It expresses what we cannot put into words, and it acts like a cathartic tool.

I'm sure you have lived through moments where music has calmed you or helped you express emotions which you wouldn't be able to express in any other way. Sometimes you might have used it to calm down in moments of stress or to encourage you when you may be suffering from pain, loss or separation.

Many of us use music as something cathartic. I remember when a friend of mine was upset and he listened to the same sad song for hours and days, it seemed like he needed to listen to music that vibrated at the same frequency of the pain he felt, and according to him, it soothed him. Music allowed him to represent what he felt and what he could not express in any other way through sound.

The opposite also happens when we are overwhelmed with happiness and we get lost in the rhythmic music turned up to the highest volume to express through the vibrations and sound the ecstasy that we feel, that feeling that goes beyond the realm of explanation, of word. Sometimes only music can express the depth of the emotions that we harbor.

In hospitals, music began to be used to treat pain after World War I in the hospitals of veterans when groups of volunteer musicians performed for soldiers who had lost limbs, were recovering from serious injuries, and also for many who had lost friends and lived through intense emotional experiences. The results of this encounter between music and pain were so grand that the field of music therapy arose and nowadays has become a profession for thousands of people. From then on, many studies have shown that music reduces stress, anxiety, depression and the pain of physical and emotional scars.

Music began to be "prescribed" for specific purposes in so-called musical interventions, where music therapists expose patients to different types of music in controlled environments once or several times a day. The "dosage" of music depends on the ailment and can be administered in one and several sessions.

To select the appropriate music, the therapists strike up a relationship with the patient to discover their tastes and associations that they have with different types of music.

Although the general belief is that the music that has a greater effect of calming pain or anxiety is Western classical music, that could not be further from the truth. This false belief has developed as the majority of studies about the use of music in clinical environments have been carried out in Western countries, where this type of music is associated culturally and socially with certain codes and sociocultural environments. Surely if we did studies in countries outside of this Western axis, we would find that every culture responds to different types of music. In other words, the use and effects of music must be culturally, socially and historically contextualized.

This requires a personalized approach for each patient, where the patient is seen in their entirety, as a bio-psycho-social being, and the patients themselves are studied, not their illness and from that point, their sound treatment can be designed. In other words, if we had to design a musical handbook, we would be faced with the challenge of creating one for each and every cultural and social environment.

Contrary to what we might think, music therapy treatments aren't just limited to listening to music. They include any type of musical activity like performing, composing, learning an instrument and singing. Music is created and experienced through the body and through it, physical and emotional pain is relieved and motor and cognitive skills are developed. The benefits of music go far beyond the relief of pain and are supported by an infinity of studies.[156,157,158]

From a physiological point of view, the relationship between pain and music is backed by *Gate Control Theory*, one of the most accepted theories about pain, developed by Melzack and Wall, who recognized the emotional and cognitive components of pain. This theory postulated that pain signals travel through the thin nerve fibers, while tactile sensations like vibration, touch or pressure travel through wide fibers. When we receive a pain stimulus, the nerve sensors send both signals to the spinal cord, which acts as a gateway to decide which of the signals should be let in, the tactile or the pain one. The most interesting and relevant thing for our relationship between music and pain is that the wide fibers, apart from processing tactile stimuli, also process auditory and visual stimuli.[159]

Gate Control Theory explains why sometimes we massage a painful area and it soothes us, in other words, the tactile stimulus of the massage competes with the pain stimulus and in essence, it gains entry to the spinal cord. Thus, what we feel is the touch of the massage, not pain.[160]

If we consider the fact that music is a multimodal experience which doesn't just impact the ear but also tactile perception through vibration, visual perception through the associations that it evokes and the emotional and cognitive spheres, we all have the elements that allow us to explain, at least empirically, the effect of music to control pain.

A more recent theory about pain, also developed by Melzack, called *Neuromatrix Theory*,[161] proposes the involvement of the limbic system and cerebral cortex in pain mechanisms, giving the phenomenon of pain an even wider and multidimensional aspect which further reinforces the relationship between music and the control of pain.

Numerous studies have shown that the involvement of music reduces the intensity and anguish related to pain, and it also reduces heat rate, blood pressure, breathing rate and the need for both opioid and non-opioid painkillers. In other words, music has a proven effect on the treatment of pain.[162]

For cancer patients, who frequently suffer from intense physical and emotional pain, numerous studies have shown that the active listening of music reduces the anxiety associated with pain and death,[163,164] reduces the severity of symptoms like nausea and vomiting associated with chemotherapy,[165] and it soothes anxiety and pain during radiotherapy.[166] Music also increases motivation, the feeling of wellness and the ability to exercise for patients with a bone marrow transplant,[167] as well as reducing pain for patients with severe burns[168] and the post-operatory pain for heart patients.[169]

Although the benefits of music at a physical level are highly important, perhaps it's psycho-social effect is even more important, in other words, its effect on emotional health and on our ability to fit in socially, to accept those changes that will inevitably befall us at some point in our lives; after all, life is just a constant adaptation to new environments, people, challenge, physical and social transformations.

One of the changes that each and every single one of us will have to face at some point in our lives is illness. When it impedes our lives, it transforms it, causing changes and losses that lead us to mourning. Illness launches a whole lot of bio-psycho-social processes which have an impact on all aspects of our daily life, affecting our habits and relationships. Illness also makes us confront our own mortality, the fact that our days have a date of expiry, and that we are not here forever. Death represents the most fundamental crisis of being.

In these moments of loss and confrontation, throughout history, music has played a very important role. In some of the first ever tombs which can be dated back to the Neolithic period, remains of harps and other musical instruments have been found, which apparently seem to be buried to accompany the deceased in their journey to the other world.[170] Similar figures have been found in the 5 BC tombs of Ancient Egypt and China. In the Egyptian tombs, musicians are playing percussion instruments, probably to keep away the bad spirits, a still-present tradition in Egypt.

Etruscan Iconography shows dancers and musicians playing the aulos, a wind instrument similar to a flute, in funeral ceremonies. This custom was maintained until Roman times when it was a requirement to have two guilds of musicians participating in all festivals, public games and funeral processions,

In the old Mesopotamia and in the near East, communal funeral songs were sung. In China, famous poetry called "*lamentations for the south*" was sung, and in Ancient Greece, funeral songs were accompanied by the three-stringed lyre. But it is perhaps in Greek mythology where we find one of the main figures in Western culture who showed the relation between music and death: Orpheus, the Sirens and the Muses.[171] Although the representations of these figures have been dated to the Helenistic era, the myth of *Orpheus* probably had its origins way back in 6 BC.

Orpheus, the one who tamed wild beasts with music, the one who could move trees and rocks and change the course of rivers just with the sound of his lyre, who dodged all the dangers of the underworld with his music in order to save his beloved Eurydice from the clutches of death.

The Sirens, birds with a human head, used music to seduce travelers in order to bring them to an island where they would meet their death, and the Muses appear in the works of Homer as musicians at Achilles' funeral, acting as guardians of the order of the cosmos and choir members during the parties of the gods. Musicians and music are there to help us pass to the other world, to protect and guide us in our journey into the unknown.

But apart from assisting the departed in their journey, music also helps to preserve the memory of the community, to have hope and move on with our lives.

In Iran, while the women cry for the deceased, the men sing and dance. In rural areas of China, el *xisang* (happy funeral) is celebrated for those who lived a long life and the *xiongsang* (unhappy funeral)[172] for those who had a short life. The atmosphere of these two types of funerals is made up of musical and aural events, including representation of folkloric music for friends and family of the dead. In the Colombian Pacific, communities of African descent sing songs called *Alabaos*, which are lively celebrations in which the whole community participates. Similarly, within the black community in New Orleans, jazz funerals are celebrated, a tradition that can be dated right back to the history of the city. In these celebrations, groups of musicians form a parade in honour of death. These rituals help the mourning process and the mental health of those closest to the deceased.[173]

In the Christian tradition, we are familiar with many musical works composed since the 16th century to accompany the Office of the Dead and to declare the existence of eternal life, an act of faith and hope for believers.

The first *Requiem* recorded was composed by Johannes Ockeghem (1461), followed by numerous works including Brumel's Requiem (1483), Jean

Richafort's Requiem for six voices, Antoine de Févin's (15th century), Tomás Luis de Victoria's (1603), just to name a few from that period. More recent and well known requiems have been composed by Mozart (1791), Cherubini (1816) Brahms (1865–68), Verdi (1874), Saint-Saëns (1878), Berlioz (1837), Faure (1887), Durufle (1947), Britten (1961) Ligetti (1963), Stravinsky (1966), Penderecki (1980–2005), Lloyd Webber (1985), Rutter (1985), Jenkins (2005), and an infinite number of compositions of Western musicians intended for the Office of the Dead.

What all of these funeral rites of the past have in common is that they aim to restore the balance of the community, which was lost due to the death of one of its members. The words of the songs, the music, the speeches and the lamentations are there to remind and preserve the memory of the deceased. Through songs and lamentations, the community is able to restore the memory, experience catharsis of pain, connect this earthly life with life beyond and preserve collective memory.

Although these rituals are directed at the dead, in reality they serve as spaces to reaffirm life, spaces of resilience where passions and emotions are exuberantly expressed through word, music and dance, with the body acting as a vehicle.

Death is without doubt one of the most important social and vital events, the only certainty that we have in our constantly changing and flowing existence. Sadly, despite its importance, in our current society we tend to deny it and glorify all representations of youth and beauty. For many people, being faced with death causes conflict and most of the time it is denied and we prefer not to talk about it, to sidestep, to believe that its something which happens to others and when it happens, it's a tragedy. Unfortunately death isn't seen as what it essentially is, a natural occurrence, a process which we will all inevitably go through and therefore, something we should be prepared for.

Music can also help prepare us for our own death and for the death of our close ones. In one study, patients who had terminal illnesses or those who had sought assisted suicide, as well as their close ones, were asked to create a playlist to listen to during death or during their last hours or days of life. Some people chose music which made them relaxed or happy, others chose songs that had a special meaning in some moment of their life, songs which reflected their values or experiences. For example, some patients made playlists which included music from their childhood, adolescence and youth, a sort of musical autobiography which ended with songs that they would like to be played during their funeral. Music helped them to build a narrative that linked their past, present and future.[174]

Projects, like the one done by *Chalice of Repose,*[175] are based on music accompanying patients with terminal illnesses and their families through musical intervention in the final days of their life and during their death. These interventions include passive and attentive listening of music and composition of songs, a very powerful exercise as by combining text and music, we reach levels of expression which you normally would not be able to access, we can express the depths of our pain, our fear, our vulnerability, our hope.

In this context, music serves as a narrator and a tool by which we release our memories and emotions, and it's as though music is an extension of our being, a part of who we are that it is expressed outside of our body and it makes us, and those who join our listening experience, vibrate. Music allows us to directly access emotions and create a narrative, an autobiography in which you make amends between your expectation of who you wanted to be and who you are in reality, in other words, we can look back on our lives and build a bridge between the real us and the idealized version of us, which helps us accept who we really are, including accepting our mortality and viewing it as a natural process.

Composing songs, even if we are not musicians, is a very powerful exercise and within everyone's reach. Why don't we compose songs for the person that we were, who we are now and who we would like to be? Why don't we write for those who we leave behind, songs to say goodbye to our loved ones, to express our gratitude or love for them or to give them hope? Why don't we start to think about the songs that would play at our funeral?

These exercises that seem superfluous are in reality very powerful confrontations with our own mortality, transformative exercises which help us to reflect about who we truly are and about the mark we want to leave on the world, about our values and about the impact that our actions have on society and the environment.

The beautiful thing about music is that it is within the reach of everybody; you don't need special musical training to create a song or enjoy a melody and reap in its positive effects on our mental and physical health.

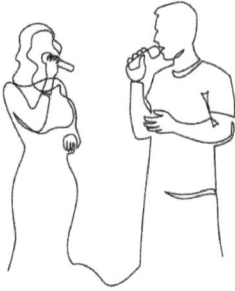

Chapter 8

VOICE, SONG AND THE SOUNDS OF THE BODY

Do you remember the tunes that your parents sang to you when you were a child to calm you down, make you happy or to guide you? Or perhaps your first school songs come to mind, those songs that you happily shared with your family and that led to family evenings together?

In our childhood, we sing and dance freely, we shout, we cry melodiously and our cries are heard far away as our breathing and vocal emission mechanisms have not yet been "tamed". We still haven't internalized the rules that determine what is correct or the valued judgment that limits us as adults when we sing and when we constantly evaluate whether we're singing well or badly or if we're making a fool of ourselves.

Singing is something inherent in human beings, in fact, when an adult begins to learn singing, the first steps are to remember and relearn the freedom and relaxation with which we made sound during our childhood. We start by learning to breathe in a completely relaxed state, conscious of our body, of our posture, relaxing our jaw muscles, our tongue, our neck, our rib cage. The process of learning to sing becomes a journey in self-awareness which has a physical component that connects us to our body, makes us conscious of it, makes us introspect, look into ourselves, be in touch with ourselves. The body is the instrument of the singer.

But perhaps the most important component when learning to sing is the emotional component. Our voice becomes the metaphor for our being, for the space of representation where part of our being is projected in the most pure and authentic manner.

Some people find it hard to listen to their own voices, they get nervous or embarrassed listening to a voice recording of themselves and they don't like what they hear. Learning to sing therefore becomes a journey of accepting ourselves, and recognising who we are, without facades or exaggerations. We are simply who we are and that is enough. We don't need to be anything else to be loved, accepted, or valued.

The process of getting used to and accepting my own voice is a process in which I get used to and accept myself. Throughout this process, I have come to love who I am. But this journey doesn't end here, as the process of learning to sing teaches us that each person's voice is unique, a digital footprint that differentiates us from others and one which is in continuous construction and development.

The study of the technical side of singing also teaches us that although we begin the journey with a *tessitura* or a vocal extension, our voice can develop to its full potential, a potential that we didn't even know we possessed. Our voice, like the rest of our body and brain, changes throughout life, mirroring the experiences and physical and emotional stages that we go through during our life cycle.

The process of taking both our real and metaphorical voice to its highest level of expression is a process of self-awareness and acceptance where we are aware of our bodies and we learn to coordinate relaxation, breathing and sound emission mechanisms in an environment of complete awareness and freedom.

Perhaps many of you are now thinking that your voice isn't beautiful, that you're not able to sing. Luckily, although we would all love to have a beautiful singing voice in line with the aesthetic ideals of our society, the act of singing transcends these ideals, and therefore we all can and must sing.

Singing is essentially communicating, giving the world a part of me, expressing my beliefs, my ideals, my dreams. The singer, while reflecting the reality around them, transcends this reality, transforming themselves. When singing, they can reach other planes of reality, forms of perception and subtle expression. In this almost magical act, they connect with that ancestral shaman and priest, and become the bridge that connects the ordinary world with the symbolic world, the ethereal, abstract and transcendent world.

Throughout history, singing has been used to heal, soothe pain, express happiness, give strength to those who are sent off to war, energize those who work long, dull hours, comfort those who are suffering, provide company to those who feel alone.

They say that Isabel of Farnesio, the second wife of the Spanish king, Felipe the 5th, invited the Napolitan castrato Carlo Broschi, the famous Farinelli to court, in order to pull the king out of his depression, as songs were the only way to rescue him from isolation and apathy. This anecdote that may seem funny can be backed up by science. Listening to happy music or music that has an emotional connection to us has proven effects on our wellbeing and mood.

A recent study by the *British Academy of Sound Therapy,*[176] using the *Oxford Happiness Questionnaire*[177], concluded that after listening to music, 32.07% of people were more prone to happiness, 64.97% felt happier, 89.31% more energetic, 64.97% laughed more, 86.31% felt more satisfied with their lives, 84.67% felt like they had a positive effect on others, 82.4% felt more in control of their lives and 80.06% said that feeling happier helped them make decisions more easily. Singing and listening to others sing has positive effects on physical and mental health.

The key part of a song is voice, that digital footprint that differentiates us from others, and it's important both when it makes noise and when it doesn't. Voice is essentially produced through vibrations of the vocal cords due to air.

As well as being a cathartic tool, songs help to convey the values of a person or of a community, as a badge of personal and social identity. This is why we identify with songs from a generation, political party or artist themselves, because songs transcend the musical aspect to become a gate to a culture, to the values and aspirations of people and nations, they are an essential part of our heritage, for both us as individuals and for our species.

Music and song in particular date back to the dawn of our species. Although proponents of musical proto-language tend to place its beginnings in evolutionary scenarios prior to 400,000 years ago, recent studies have shown that from an evolutive standpoint, the ability to produce complex vocalizations appears 400,000 years ago, as both Homo Sapiens and Neanderthals, and by extension, their last common ancestor, have the same anatomical adaptations when it comes to speech, while previous species were likely different. According to these findings, we can assume that speech and language are at least 400,000 years old and probably developed together in a process where cognitive and anatomical adaptations coevolved in a gradual manner. There is also a process of coevolution between vocalizations, gestures and communication skills; and between culture and biology, all linked by self-organization.[178]

Music and song are related to biological and adaptive processes in different species. Just like the human language, the sounds made by animals carry a lot of meaning, they express information about territories, reproduction, social groups, alliances, predation, dangers and resources. For example, the songs of birds have communicative, adaptive and reproductive purposes[179] they're used to woo their partner, to define territory and to stand out in a group. Chimpanzees adjust their sounds depending on the social group they're in and the male species of the South African clawed frog (Xenopus laevis) produces a song as part of their reproductive rites.[180] Their song is possibly due to complex adaptive processes where there are an infinity of hormones and neuromodulator substances at work. Their larynx has androgen receptors which allow it to grow eight times more than that female of the species so that they can sing.

When it comes to humans, the first social interactions are of a musical nature. When the mother sings and whispers sweet melodies to the newborn child, hormones, such as oxytocin and vasopressin[181] sre released which are essential for the development of the social brain which fosters attachment, trust and affection between mother and child. The newborn's attraction to the familiar sound of the voice and song of their mother has an impact on their central psychological responses, like for example, the secretion of cortisol.[182]

Visual and auditory perception develop in parallel, complement each other and are just as important as each other for our development. As Sterne says:

Hearing is spherical, vision is directional; hearing immerses its subject, vision offers a perspective; sound comes to us, but vision travels to its object; hearing is concerned with interiors, vision is concerned with surfaces; hearing involves physical contact with the outside world, vision requires distance from it; hearing places you inside an event, seeing gives you perspective on an event; hearing is a primarily temporal sense, vision is a primarily spatial sense.[183]

Although we have evidence that through hearing we can get to know and understand reality in a more complete way and sometimes in a faster way than through sight, our society favours the sense of sight.

It is paradoxical given that gestures, languages and sound, all essential skills for social integration and belonging to a community, seem to have arisen through adaptation, almost at the same time, to help us survive.

This situation has mainly arisen due to the fact that in Westen culture, for centuries, especially since the Enlightenment, great narratives were constructed through the written word. From then on, humanities and sciences have distanced themselves away from tradition and folklore, legitimizing themselves through the written word, while oral tradition is associated with premodern, remote, backwards societies, and this caused the audible sphere to be demoted to second place. Sciences began to use the eye of the scientist as a reference point. And from then on we have lived in a vision-centric society.

Before the 19th century, sound was studied exclusively as language or music, idealizing music and linking it to God and to the harmony of the universe. When the concept of frequency was popularized in the 19th century, a concept previously developed by those such as Decartes or Bernoulli, sounds began to be studied as a form of vibration, giving rise to the physics, acoustics, otology and physiology that would later be developed from the 19th century onwards. In a way, the sphere of hearing was legitimized once it began to enter the scientific rationalist discussion.

In medicine, just like in philosophy, vision is studied over hearing. According to Sterne, this was partly due to the difficulty to access the miniscule structures of the ear and the difficulty to study them in human bodies, something only normalized from the mid-19th century onwards when doctors finally were allowed to carry out the dissection of cadavers and were able to observe these structures.[184]

Medical semiology, one of the most valuable bodies of knowledge within medical practice, which gives doctors the tools to observe in order to diagnose complex pathologies, was mainly developed based on visual observation. Thanks to the study of semiology, doctors diagnose by observing posture, way of walking, colour of the skin, breathing rate, eyes, movement and an endless number of physical and psychological characteristics. Although semiology also deals with sound phenomena, such as heart rate, breathing rate or timber of the voice, the majority of our evaluation is visual.

However, it was a tool for listening which became one of the key elements for the professionalization of medicine. From the incorporation of the stethoscope onwards, medicine went from being purely theoretical to being perceptual. Examining the patient using sound equipment, listening and interpreting the sounds of the body became a necessity for doctors.

Although Hippocrates had already written about the important of immediate auscultation, which consisted of putting the ear directly on the body of the patient, and in 1761, in his *Inventum novum*,[185] Leopold Auenbrugger advocated for the use of percussion, which required interpretation of the sounds produced by the percussion in specific areas of the body, before the invention of the stethoscope and audio examining (through the means of an instrument), the doctor exclusively depended on visual observation and the patient's narration to draw up the diagnosis. The voice of the patient, their narration and visual observation were the most important pillars of information for the diagnosis.

From the incorporation of the stethoscope onwards, and the development of the ability to link certain sounds in the body, picked up by the stethoscope, to illnesses, the internal sounds of the body became the most important source of information for diagnosis and voice began to be important for its timbral qualities, in other words, being analyzed based on the type of sound it produces.

In 1816, when Rene Laennec wrote that he could hear the sounds of a patient's heart better while listening through a rolled up cylinder of paper over the chest, his innovation didn't exactly lead to the invention of the tube itself, but rather to the ability to link the sounds of the body, the internal organs, to possible illnesses. From this moment on, a series of observations began which culminated in the publication of his *Treaty on mediate auscultation,*[186] a founding work in which, for the first time, auscultated sound was linked to disease of the lung, heart and thoracic cavity.

Listening became essential for doctors and the stethoscope allowed them to listen to what they could not see. Sounds became signals which indicated good health or illness, and doctors thought it necessary to refine the sense of hearing, to develop auditory skills for scientific purposes, and the sphere of hearing was made rational.

The sounds of the body have also had a long relationship with music and the arts. The heartbeat, the rhythmic sounds that have been a metaphor for love throughout history, the emotions and life, were described for the first time by the Greek doctor Praxagoras of Kis (340 BC) and later by Erasistrus (304-250 BC). However, it was Herophilos (335-280 BC) who deduced that the pulse was a result of the contraction and dilation of the arteries, being the first person to reference its musical qualities.

His theories, which bestowed the pulse with a musical metric, had a considerable impact on musical creation during the Middle Ages and the Renaissance, when people such as Boethius (480-524 AD) distinguished between three types of music: *musica mundana,* which comes from the celestial spheres, *musica humana,* caused by the pulse, breathing and heartbeat and *musica instrumentis,* the only type of music that humans can hear.[187]

From then on, the heart became a common theme in art, being associated with love, kindness and other Christian values. From the 20th century onwards, thanks to digital technology, the heartbeat was used to create interactive artistic works which connected body, emotion, creativity and music. A recent example is the *Heart Chamber Orchestra*, an audiovisual spectacle made up of 12 classical musicians and the artistic duo *Terminalbeach*. Linking the heartbeats to a composition and visualization software in real time, musicians can interpret sheet music made by their own hearts.[188] The creation of this orchestra is an example of the so-called biometric art, which is based on the sounds and shapes of the body to make art, a true fusion of knowledge which reflects the interdisciplinarity which we are returning to in the 21st century. Biometric analysis allows us to create music based on data taken from the body, but it also opens the door to make medical diagnosis easier.

Taking advantage of the sensitivity we have as humans to distinguish variations in sound, biochemists at Michigan State University invented the analysis of musical urine,[189] a type of research that allows, for example, doctors with a visual disability to analyse the results, just like those who are performing a surgery and who don't have their hands or eyes free. Musical analysis allows a high specificity because humans are more sensitive to variations in tone than to numerical variations. This caused the geneticist Susumo Ohno to turn DNA sequences into their musical equivalents, allowing him to discover genetic patterns that would have been difficult to find any other way.[190,191]

The body is literally a symphony, a set of sounds that we can now listen to thanks to experiments which turn our electric signals and muscle movements into music by using a simple electronic instrument called the *Biomuse.*[192]

Digiti Sonus, an artistic system that turns digital footprints into sound also shows that our bodies are music. The system uses algorithms so the audience can explore their sonic identities through unique sounds generated by the patterns of their fingerprint. The most interesting thing about this is that the participants can alter the sounds, experimenting with their sound identities.[193] According to Yoon Chung Han: "given the system's ability to locate the sound in the 3D space, it is likely that the sonification of fingerprints can be used as an effective method to represent complex biometric data".[194]

Yoon Chung Han and Byeong-jun Han have also experimented with turning the many patterns and qualities of the skin into sound, in what they call sonification of the skin. The artists split up the body into its different parts: head, neck, arms, legs, chest and pelvis. In order to sonify the numerous qualities of the skin, they used an algorithm to take an average of the pixels of color specific to each part of the body and then they assigned this average color to a default range of frequency. Like this, someone could explore the skin from their whole body and examine the different sonic representations.

These experiments open the doors to a myriad of possibilities for the future and allow us to explore our bodies in different ways than we have ever done before. Soon we'll be able to listen to the sound of our skin, eyes, hands, hair and I'm sure we will also be able to distinguish between the sounds of health and sickness. This technology could also lead to endless therapeutic possibilities. If organs can sound different in health and in sickness, why not consider changing the sonic frequencies of the sick organs so that they sound like healthy ones?

If, as shown by Pelling, Gralla and Gimzewski,[195] cells can sing, who says that we can't make cells vibrate at the frequency of health? The possibilities are endless!

Sounds themselves, of both the individual and the environment, define who we are and they place us in the socio-historical context. We can create music from the sounds of the body and also from the sounds of our surrounding environment. The act of listening to ourselves and to the surroundings is in itself therapeutic, it connects us to our environment, it anchors us in the here and now. By listening, we open ourselves up to the world, we direct our attention to one another, and we begin a relationship with the exterior. As Gadamer says, "anyone who listens is fundamentally open. Without such openness there is no genuine human bond. Belonging together always means being able to listen to one another".[196]

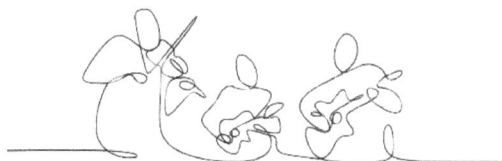

Chapter 9

MUSIC AND CREATIVITY

One of the first things we think about when we hear the words music and creativity is the composer. They have the ability to create music which represents and unravels the values, desires and fears of a society in a specific moment of history, and they turn their emotions and experiences into sounds that are chock-full of meaning.

How are they able to create works which entire generations can identify with? Are they geniuses, gifted with exceptional talent? Special people?.

In Ancient Greece, it was believed that those who took part in activities or produced output that we would

117

now consider creative were possessed by a spirit or inspired by the muses.[197] During the Middle Ages, creativity was considered a gift of God, coming from divine inspiration.[198] In the Romantic period, creativity was attributed to super gifted humans, people who were special in some way.

Research started in the 20th century revealed that creativity is within the reach of everyone, and that the great creative achievements in the fields of arts, sciences or sports weren't solely due to talent or genius; they were mainly a result of perseverance, studying and years worth of practice. Nobody has put it better than Pablo Picasso when he said "Inspiration exists, but it has to find you working."

Defined as an individual's ability to produce something new, original, suitable and valuable for a specific task, creativity is often associated with individuals[199] in other words, we tend to believe that innovation comes exclusively from the brain of a creative individual. However, creativity, like cognition, is also a sociocultural phenomenon, given that the output of the creative process is used by, appreciated, rejected or incorporated into the society in which it is created. This means that creativity isn't just limited to an individual, but rather it's a process which extends to the environment in which the individual develops their ideas.

Although there are personality traits that are more frequently associated with creative subjects, like, for example, extroversion, willingness to take risks[200] or seek out new experiences,[201] creativity also depends on factors such as habits, motivation and the conditions of our surrounding environment. This means that we can develop it, and we can cultivate habits and create environments which stimulate it.

Although we might think that creativity is a solely human characteristic, it can be found extensively in the animal kingdom.[202] Hinde and Fischer described how in order to survive, a species of bird in the UK learned to make holes in the aluminium caps of the bottles of milk left at the door, a practice that started in one area and became the norm in most of the country.[203]

According to Wallas,[204] during creative processes, there are conscious and unconscious factors involved that develop at different stages. In order to create, we have to go through a phase of preparation and acquisition of knowledge that continues the incubation of the idea. Then we arrive at that awaited moment of enlightenment, when innovation takes place. In the final stage, the idea is tested and validated.

The unconscious plays a very important role in

creativity. Many composers and creators from all fields have told us how their ideas appeared, how they sprung out from nowhere, as if someone was controlling it. I personally get surprised sometimes when I'm composing songs, as ideas come to me so quickly, in an almost magical, mysterious way.

When I compose, I usually put music to poems by famous authors and I've always found it strange how sometimes when I'm reading the poetry, suddenly I come across one poem that inspires music in my head. It's as though the music is jumping out of the page. And this phenomenon only happens with some poems, not all.

In 1997, when Karlheinz Stockhausen was asked what is intuition, he answered:

Intuition transforms every normal action into something special that one doesn't know oneself. So I am a craftsman, I can start working with sounds, with apparatuses and find all sorts of new combinations. But when I want to create something that amazes me and moves me, I need intuition. … something happens every now and then which is amazing and which is also for me unknown. Intuition comes, according to my own experience, from a higher world.[205]

The composer Pierre Boulez said that the

fundamental components of creativity are imagination and intelligence: "creative processes can't exist without imagination, but they also can't exist without training the skills to create".

When the composer Lucas Foss was asked the definition of an idea, he answered: "an idea occurs when there is chaos and suddenly you see relationships, when you find meaning where you looked before and there seemed to only be disorder".[206]

What Foss was referring to was *divergent thinking*, a type of thinking that comes up with creative ideas through exploration of many possible solutions. It is a type of thinking that, in contrast to logical thinking which looks for the one correct answer based on previous knowledge, usually happens spontaneously, fluidly, which allows many ideas to emerge in a short amount of time, connecting things in an unexpected way.

This explains why when he had a difficult problem to solve, Einstein would shut himself in and play the violin, an instrument he played since he was six years old. The physicist even stated that his famous theory of relativity came to him through intuition and that its discovery was a result of musical perception.[207]

The famous Italian composer, Edgar Varese, stated that his inspiration came from maths and astronomy because they stimulated his imagination and gave him the impression of movement and rhythm. Son of an engineer, from a young age, Varese studied in a school which specialized in maths and science. Here he discovered Leonardo da Vinci and became interested in the study of sound.

> "When I was around 20, I found a definition of music that changed my life. Józef Maria Hoene-Wroński, Polish physicist, musicologist and philosopher from the first half of the 19th century, defined music as "the corporealization of the intelligence that is in sounds". It was this definition that first made me think of music as something spatial, as bodies of sound moving in space, a conception that I gradually made my own.".[208]

From a physics point of view, music, and by extension all sounds, are viewed as energy that vibrates through a medium and is transferred to our body and senses.[209] The vibration activates our auditory system, touch[210] and the vestibular system in the inner ear. From the moment in which we perceive sound, we assign it an aesthetic value, we situate it culturally and we classify it as music or noise, as beautiful or ugly.

The history of music is intimately linked to physics. It has been said that when Einstein got to know of the quantum theory proposed by Max Planck, who won the

Nobel Prize for physics in 1918 and was also a gifted pianist and cellist, he stated that it was "the highest form of musicality in the sphere of thinking".

We could cite hundreds of examples of scientists-cum-musicians and musicians-cum-scientists who provided us with massive contributions throughout history, all thanks to an education which allowed them to develop divergent thinking.

According to Root-Bernstein, this is an example of *correlative talents*, that is to say, skills or abilities in different fields that can be merged together to produce surprising and innovative results.[211]

Creative thinking is transdisciplinary by nature and can be transferred from one field to another. The skills associated with music, like the training and recognition of patterns, synesthetic skills, imagination, aesthetic sensitivity, rhythm, the ability to interpret and express emotions and the understanding of music itself, all united by the discipline required in the field, have been important components of the correlative talents of famous scientists.[212]

The doctor Hector Berlioz (1803-1969) found worldwide fame as one of most innovative composers of the 19th century. Aleksandr Borodin (1833-1987), respected medic, chemist and founder of the St

Petersburg Women's Medical School, was also one of the greatest Russian composers throughout history, a member of the *Group of Five*.[213] Virginia Apgar, a doctor from the USA who was a reputed anesthesiologist, obstetrician and creator of the Apgar Score, a test carried out on all newborn babies to evaluate their neurological health, played the violin from a young age and learned how to build instruments. Camille Saint-Saëns (1835-1921), apart from being a composer, was also an avid astronomer. Edward Elgar (1857-1934), isn't just famous as a composer, but was also a chemist with many registered patents. The Anglo-German astronomer William Hershel (1738-1822), who discovered the planet Uranus, had a noteworthy career as a composer and helped his sister Caroline Hershel (1850-1948) to first establish herself as a singer and later as an astronomer. Caroline discovered a number of comets and was a pioneer in many ways, as she was the first woman to receive a salary as a scientist and the first woman to be accepted as a member of the Royal Astronomical Society. The famous guitarist and composer Brian May, part of the band Queen, is a doctor of astrophysics with numerous publications in the field.

The cardiologist and composer Richard Bing has said that his discoveries were a result of the transdisciplinary education he received. Nobel Prize winners, like the neuroanatomist-cum-visual artist Santiago Ramón y Cajal, and the immunologist-cum-novelist Charles Richet, have stated that the big advances that have taken place in science aren't due to monothematic specialists, but rather to people with a wide range of interests and hobbies.[214]

There is a need to develop hobbies, to promote the study of music and arts, not just as a secondary subject, but as the main one, recognizing that it is essential for cognitive and creative development. This statement can be verified by numerous studies carried out on thousands of students gifted in the field of science and maths which showed that the most important factors predicting their professional success weren't what we would expect, i.e. their IQ or academic results. The determining factors were whether they took part in cognitively challenging activities in their free time or not.[215]

With so much evidence, I once again would like to invite you, dear reader, to fill your life with music, to brighten all the aspects of your daily life with sounds, to learn an instrument and to sing. We can develop skills and environments that stimulate creative and innovative thinking, and live a fuller and healthier life. Pay attention to the sounds in your surroundings, walk around with your ears open, listen to the birds chirping, to the trees swaying in the wind, to your neighbors singing, to the music you come across during your daily strolls. Take note of your surroundings, prepare your senses for creativity. When you're having a mental block or you feel tired, stop for a minute, listen to music, take a deep breath, dance. If you are a musician, improvise, leave aside the sheet music for a second and explore the sounds of your instrument.

Cognition and creative processes interact with the surroundings, they become embodied, meaning that the environment in which you live and the habits that you develop manifest themselves in your ways of thinking and in your creative being.

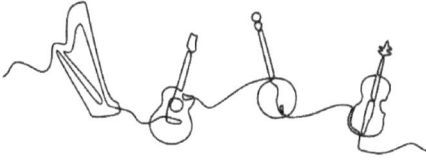

Chapter 10

GLOBAL HEALTH, PANDEMIC AND THE EXAMPLE OF ORCHESTRAS

There is no better example of working in a team or managing diversity than how an orchestra, choir, theatre or musical group works. These represent the perfect metaphor for how society should function. Every instrument, every member of the choir has a unique voice, a digital print, a stamp of their identity, however, despite differences in the forms and sounds of the instruments, each of them join to play a piece, each one bringing to the table what makes them unique, listening to others, following a rhythm and a shared melody, all united by a common goal. What each person does affects the global result.

Defining health is a very complex matter, and sometimes we fall into the trap of thinking we are healthy if we don't feel any pain, if we aren't taking medication or if we don't visit the doctor. We usually fall into the trap of thinking health is an individual concept, something which happens to me, disconnected from our surroundings. This individualist view of health is a reflection of the values of a society in which we are all competing with one another, where there is the survival of the fittest; as long as I am well, who cares about the rest.

This manner of thinking can be seen at every level, from governments that watch over their borders and implement protectionist policies which only benefit themselves, without caring about the disastrous consequences it has on other parts of the world, the methods of production that seriously harm the environment, the selling of weapons and drugs that wipe out millions of humans, high and low level corruption, our daily consumption habits, our diets, the way we dress, how we travel. It is difficult to find an area of human existence that isn't tainted by this capitalist individualism. Our health and our own body, being the first territory we have access to and control over, are no exception.

In order to understand health and sickness, we must have a holistic view of things, which links the individual and their physical and emotional aspects to their surrounding ecosystem and their cultural and social environment. In other words, health and wellbeing can only be achieved when there is a bio-psycho-social equilibrium which acknowledges the individual and their surrounding environment as inseparable, dependent on one another.

One of the most recent pieces of evidence of this individualist - I'd go so far as to say egotistical - concept of health has been the reaction to the COVID-19 pandemic, which we are living through at the time of writing this book. Thanks to the incredible advances in sciences and communication, during this pandemic - the most recent version of a long series of similar ones that humans have lived through since records have been kept - the mechanisms of transmission and the measures of containment of the virus were quickly identified, with this information very quickly reaching most of the world population. We recognized that measures as simple as using a mask or washing hands were critical to contain the spreading of the virus.

One of the greatest learnings during the pandemic has been that our actions have repercussions on the life and health of the people around us. Our habits directly impact the health of our neighbors, our friends, the people in our country, in the world, on the planet. The lesson to be taken out of all this is that this situation isn't just limited to the transmission of a virus, it extends to all areas of life.

Although the conclusion seems obvious, during the pandemic we are seeing that despite the evidence, millions of people around the world are not following these preventative measures. Interviews with people who don't wear a mask or break the rules show that they believe they are simply exercising their right to freedom, and that they're doing nothing wrong because ultimately it's their own life they are risking: "if I get sick, it's my problem, not anyone else's". This way of analyzing the situation reflects an individualist concept of sickness that places me at the centre, a me which is isolated and disconnected from my environment.

In contrast, the individual that sees themselves as part of a community knows that their actions and habits will impact those around them, their environment, their community, their country, their planet, and they are aware of this social impact on both a local scale and a global one.

How can we internalize correctly from childhood this social conscience when we live in a world that promotes individualism? Music and art are once again the answer.

There are many examples where participation in artistic activities has been successfully used to mobilize communities, include and empower marginalized groups, educate people about issues related to health or to raise awareness about healthy practices. As tools of representation of the values of the community, arts are critical for the education and health of individuals and the community at a global scale.

From a public health point of view, the pandemic has also led governments to a long overdue paradigm shift, which transcends the interests of the local community, and cares about making sure every town in the world is equipped to deal with it and has access to healthcare. The need for herd immunity to be able to force this pandemic out has made rich countries recognize the need to help poorer ones, not as an act of generosity or charity but rather as a crucial step for their own public health. It means nothing to be a rich country with the whole population vaccinated if one part of the world isn't, as the virus still would not have gone away.

We've moved away from the paradigm of "public health", in which policies are made focusing on topics affecting the health of local communities of cities and countries, onto the paradigm of "global health", based on issues that transcend national borders, and directly or indirectly affect the health of communities.

Achieving a global health paradigm that aims to secure an equal and fair access to healthcare, requires a high level of cooperation between governments. Due to its complexity, this global health paradigm crucially requires a transdisciplinary approach that goes beyond the sciences of health.

By recognizing that health and sickness are also cultural concepts, a global approach views the humanities and arts as indispensable tools. There will no longer be arrogant public health interventions in which a member of the health system goes to a community to teach or impose measures which are completely out of context or incoherent with the people and their territories. We are working towards an ecological approach, which recognizes the relationship between the individual, their social context and their surrounding environment.

In this context, music, apart from its positive effects on personal and collective health, serve as a resource for individuals and their communities to build habits, express civil unrest, mend relationships within the community, bring together different generations and in general, promote physical and emotional health. If we look at it this way, music is an essential part of the ecosystem of health, fundamental for the development of the individual and community at a local and global level.

Understanding this should be enough to incorporate music and arts into the lives of every person, as well as into government policy. This understanding should suffice for budgets given to arts and humanities to be just as important as those given to the sciences. It should be enough for the government to start campaigns to encourage the participation of boys in arts and humanities, in contrast to the current climate which pushes women into STEM. We should celebrate the fact that girls show interest in the arts rather than discourage them. Understanding that music is vital for health should be enough for access to musical education and expression to be seen as a right, as promulgated by the International Music Council in their *Five Music Rights*.

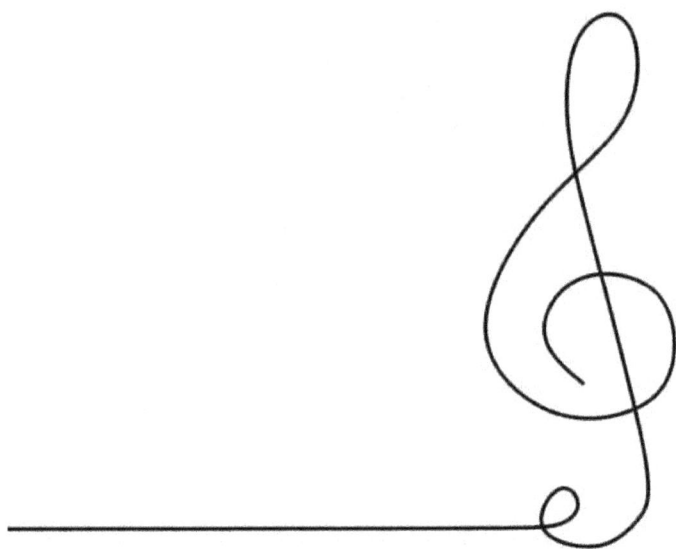

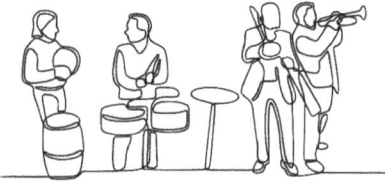

EXERCISE BOOK

I hope that after having read this book and understood the importance of music for your physical, emotional and social health, you're ready to take action and incorporate it into your life, and consciously use it as a tool to improve your health and make you feel happier.

Therefore, in this section, I invite you to complete some exercises based on some of the studies I based my research on. Come reflect about the role of music in your life, create playlists with your favourite songs or with music you associate with different moods. These exercises will help you understand yourself better, discover who you once were and who you will become, prepare you for your death and the death of your loved ones. I'm sure you'll also have fun doing these exercises, so let's get going!

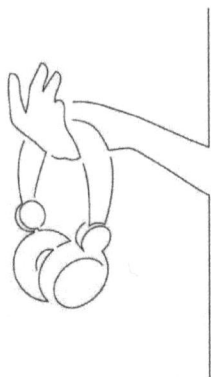

1

THE SOUNDTRACK OF YOUR LIFE

Autobiographical exercise

In this section, I invite you to reflect on the music that has accompanied you throughout your life. Right from your childhood to the present day, let's make a note of the music that is linked to your history, your dreams and your beliefs. At the end of the section, I also invite you to create a Spotify playlist with your favourite music and share it on social media with the hashtag *#wearewhatwelistento*

A. Write down the most important songs from your childhood.

_____

_____

_____

_____

_____

_____

_____

B. Write down the music of your adolescence, the songs or soundtracks that marked this stage of your life.

.

_____

_____

_____

_____

_____

_____

_____

_____

C. Write down the songs that have accompanied you in your sad moments.

.

_____

_____

_____

_____

_____

D. Write down the songs that have accompanied you in the happy moments of your life, or the music that makes you feel happy.

.

_____

_____

_____

_____

_____

_____

E. Write down the songs that make you feel most relaxed, that help bring you to inner peace with yourself.

.

_____

_____

_____

_____

_____

_____

F. Write down the songs that you will pass on to your children and grandchildren or to the young people you love.

_____

_____

_____

_____

_____

_____

G. Write down the music that you'd like in your funeral

_____

_____

_____

_____

_____

H. Write down the ten songs that have accompanied you in the most important moments of your life and explain why each one is important. Create a playlist on Spotify or Youtube with your favourite versions of each.

1._____

_____

_____

2._____

_____

_____

3._____

_____

_____

4._____

_____

_____

5._____

_____

_____

6._____

_____

_____

7._____

_____

_____

8._____

_____

_____

9._____

_____

_____

10._____

_____

_____

Remember, share your playlists on social media with the hashtag
#wearewhatwelistento

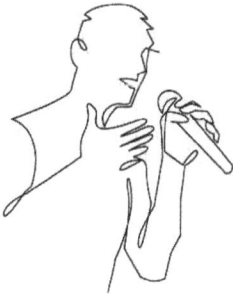

2

CREATION EXERCISE
Your essence in music

The creation or composition of songs is within the reach of everyone. You don't have to be a professional musician to write a text which reflects who you are, your beliefs, aspirations, dreams, sadness, losses and desires. This creation exercise is an invitation to reflect upon the beliefs and qualities that define you, and is also an opportunity to ponder over who you want to become, the habits you want to develop, the bonds you want to strengthen.

This autobiographical exercise is very powerful, and through it, we can come to terms with who we are, forgive ourselves and even prepare ourselves for our death and that of our loved ones.

CREATE SONGS THAT EXPRESS YOUR ESSENCE

A. Write a song which expresses your beliefs and your outlook on life.

._____

_____

_____

_____

_____

_____

_____

_____

_____

_____

_____

_____

_____

_____

_____

B. Write a song in which you describe the person you want to become.

_____

_____

_____

_____

_____

_____

_____

_____

_____

_____

_____

_____

_____

_____

_____

_____

_____

_____

_____

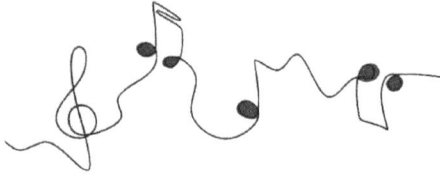

3

SOUNDSCAPES

The sounds of your everyday life

We are immersed in a sea of sounds. Although usually we ignore them, we encounter the voices of others, the sounds of cars, the birds, the wind, the cries of street vendors, the metro, sirens, the conversations of people on the street, our home appliances, the noises of animals on a regular basis. Our surrounding environment makes noise, and even when we think we're in silence, in the background, there is a gentle gust of wind, a chirping of crickets, a rustling of leaves on a tree, a swishing of waves in the sea. The sounds of our surrounding environment affect our mood, usually in ways we are not even aware of, but that are ever-present. This exercise aims to make you aware of this reality and to help you foster healthy soundscapes. It also aims to make you aware that the sounds of a place are its fingerprints, its hallmark, not just every person, but every place in the world and every moment in history has its own sound.

A. Your everyday sounds

_____

_____

_____

_____

_____

_____

_____

_____

_____

_____

B. The sounds of your city

_____

_____

_____

_____

_____

_____

_____

C. The sounds of your favourite natural landscape

_____

_____

_____

_____

_____

_____

_____

Remember, share your music and experiences on social media with the hashtag #wearewhatwelistento and follow Patricia Caicedo on Spotify where you will find hundreds of playlists.

Follow her on Instagram as well at @patriciacaicedobcn

BIBLIOGRAPHY

1. Three initiates, (2009). *The Kybalion*: *A Study of the Hermetic Philosophy of Ancient Egypt*. Mineola,New York: Dover Publications Inc.

2.Requena Rodríguez, A. (2008). "Nada está inmovil; todo se mueve; todo vibra". Academia de Ciencias de la Región de Murcia, Internet [https://www.um.es/acc/nada-esta-inmovil-todo-se-mueve-todo-vibra/]. Consultado 5 de mayo, 2020.

3. Pelling AE, Sehati S, Gralla EB, Valentine JS, Gimzewski JK. (2004). "Local nanomechanical motion of the cell wall of Saccharomyces cerevisiae", *Science*. 2004 Aug 20;305 (5687):1147-50.

4.Reuters (2020). "Coronavirus, the musical" en Medscape. Internet [https://www.medscape.com/viewarticle/929061]. Consultado 3 de mayo, 2020.

5. Darwin, C. (1872). *The expression of the emotions in man and animals*. London: John Murray.

6. Steven Mithen (2005). *The Singing Neanderthals: The Origins of Music, Language, Mind, and Body*. Cambridge: Harvard University Press.

7.Levitin, D. (2008). *The World in Six Songs: How the Musical Brain Created Human Nature*. New York: Dutton/Penguin and Toronto: Viking/Penguin.

8.Roosth, Sophia. (2009) "Screaming Yeast: Sonocytology, Cytoplasmic Milieus, and Cellular Subjectivities." *Critical Inquiry*, vol. 35, no. 2: 332–350. JSTOR, www.jstor.org/stable/10.1086/596646.

9. Pelling AE, Sehati S, Gralla EB, Valentine JS, Gimzewski JK. (2004). "Local nanomechanical motion of the cell wall of Saccharomyces cerevisiae", *Science*. 2004 Aug 20;305 (5687):1147-50.

10. Begouëm, M. y Breul, H. (1934). "De quelques figures hybrides (mi-humaines et mianimales) de la caverne des Trois-Frères (Ariège)." *Revue Anthropologique,* vol. XLIV, n° 4-6, p. 115-119.

11.Vitebski, P. (1996). *The Shaman: Voyages of the Soul. Trance, Ecstasy and Healing from Siberia*. Macmillan and Duncan Baird Publishers.

12. Sibbing Plantholt, I. (2017). "The image of divine healers: Healing goddesses and the legitimization of the Asû in the Mesopotamian Medical Marketplace". Ph.D. Diss. University of Pennsylvania.

13. Aristotle. *Politics in The Complete Works of Aristotle*: *The Revised Oxford Translation*, ed. Jonathan Barnes, 2 vols. Princeton, NJ: Princeton University Press, 1983, Book VIII, 1338b 1, 2122.

14.West, M. (2000). "Music Therapy in Antiquity," in *Music as Medicine: The History of Music Therapy Since Antiquity*, ed. Peregrine Horden. Burlington, VT: Ashgate Publishing Limited, 56.

15. Portnoy, J. (1954). *The Philosopher and Music: A Historical Outline*. New York: The Humanities Press: 8.

16. Porfirio (1987). *Vida de Pitágoras ; Argonáuticas órficas ; Himnos órficos*. Introducción y traducción Miguel Periago Lorente. Gredos. Madrid. 1987.

17. Istambouli, M.N. (1981). 'The history of Arabic Medicine based on the work of Ibn Abi Usaybeiah 1203 - 270". Ph.D. Diss. Loughborough University of Technology.

18. Khan, Hazrat. I. (1996). *The Mysticism of Sound and Music. The Sufi Teaching of Azrat Inayat Khan*. Boston: Shambhala Dragon Editions, 9.

19. Salmen, W. (1980) "Geisslerlieder", in *The New Grove Dictionary of Music and Musicians*, ed. Stanley Sadie. 20 vol. London: Macmillan Publishers Ltd.

20. Ficino, M. (1980). *The Book of Life*, trans. Charles Boer. Dallas: Spring Publications, Inc.,1980.

21. Voss, A. (2002). "Marsilio Ficino, the Second Orpheus," en *Music as Medicine: The History of Music Therapy Since Antiquity*, ed. Peregrine Horden. Burlington, VT: Ashgate Publishing Limited, 155.

22. Zarlino, G. (1998). "Istitutioni harmoniche", en *Source Readings in Music History*, ed. Oliver Strunk. New York: W.W. Norton Company, 294.

23. IBID, 296.

24. Hall, S.K. (2017) "The Doctrine of Affections: Where Art Meets Reason," *Musical Offerings*: Vol. 8 : No. 2 , Article 2.

25. Fink, H.J. (1953). "The Doctrine of Affections and Handel: The Background, Theory, and Practice of the Doctrine of Affections With a Comprehensive Analysis of the Oratorios of G.F.Handel". PhD diss., Western Reserve University: 116.

26. Bertrand, A. "Descartes's Compendium of Music," *Journal of the History of Ideas* 26, No. 1 (Jan-March 1965): 128-129.

27. Gouk, P. (2004), "Raising Sprits and Restoring Souls: Early Modern Medical Explanations for Music's Effects," in *Hearing Cultures: Essays on Sound, Listening and Modernity*, ed. Veit Erlmann. New York: Berg Publishers, 92.

28. Monk, E. S. (2010). A Case for Music as Therapy: "Healing and Purgation," and the Expressiveness of Music from Antiquity through the Eighteenth Century. Bachelor of Arts Diss. Presbyterian College.

29. Agrawal,S. R. (2005) "'Tune thy Temper to these Sounds': Music and Medicine in the English Ayre". PhD diss., Northwestern University, 30.

30. Gouk, P. (2002). "Sister Disciplines? Music and Medicine in Historical Perspective." In *musical Healing in Cultural Contexts*. Burlington, VT: Ashgate Publishing Limited.

31. Alvin, J. (1966). *Music Therapy*. New York: Basic Books Inc.

32. Browne, R. (1728). *Medicina Musica: A mechanical essay on singing, musick and dancing containing their uses and abuses; and demonstrating, by clear evident reasons, the alterations they produce in a human body*. London: J. Pemberton, 1727: 2.

33. Brocklesby, R. (1749). *Reflections on ancient and modern music, with the application to the cure of diseases. To which is subjoined, an essay to solve the questions, wherein consisted the difference of antient musick, from that of modern times*. London: M. Cooper, 1.

34. https://www.musictherapy.org/about/history/

35. O'Neill Kane, E. (1914). "Phonograph in operating-room", J*ournal of the American Medical Association*, vol.62, no.23, p. 1829.

36. Burdick, W. P. (1915). "The use of music during anesthesia and analgesia". in F. H. McMechan (Ed.), *The American year-book of anesthesia & analgesia*. New York: Surgery Publishing Company: 164- 167.

37. Bernardi L, Porta C, Sleight P. (2006). "Cardiovascular, cerebrovascular, and respiratory changes induced by different types of music in musicians and non-musicians: the importance of silence." In *Heart* 92: 445- 452

38. Levin, T. and Edgerton, M. E. (1999). "The Throat Singers of Tuva", *Scientific American*, September, 80-87.

39. Levin, T. (2019). *Where Rivers and Mountains Sing: Sound, Music, and Nomadism in Tuva and Beyond.* Indiana University Press.

40. Simonett, H. 2014. "Envisioned, Ensounded, Enacted: Sacred Ecology and Indigenous Musical Experience in Yoreme Ceremonies of Northwest Mexico." *Ethnomusicology* 58 (1): 110–132.

41. Schlaug, G. (2008). *Music, Musicians, and Brain Plasticity.* Oxford Handbooks. Online. Web.

42. Leeds, J. (2010). *The power of sound: How to be healthy and productive using music and sound.* Rochester, VT: Healing Arts Press.

43. Rieger, A. (2016). "Crossmodal cognition". Doctoral Diss. Dartmouth College.

44. Sagiv, N., & Frith, C. D. (2013). *Synesthesia and Consciousness.* Oxford Handbooks Online.

45. Cytowic, Richard E. (2002). *Synesthesia: A Union of the Senses.* Cambridge, MA: A Bradford Book.

46. Triarhou, L. C. (2016). "Neuromusicology or Musiconeurology? "Omni-art" in Alexander Scriabin as a Fount of Ideas". *Frontiers in Pshycology.* Vol.7, Article 364, March 2016.

47. Köhler, W. (1929). *Gestalt Psychology.* New York: Liveright.

48. Sievers, B. & Polansky, L. & Casey, M. & Wheatley, T. (2012). "Music and movement share a dynamic structure that supports universal expressions of emotion". *Proceedings of the National Academy of Sciences of the United States of America.* 110. 10.1073/pnas.1209023110.

49. Verhaeghen, P. (2011). "Aging and Executive Control: Reports of a Demise Greatly Exaggerated." *Curr Dir Psychol Sci*, 20(3), 174-180. doi:10.1177/0963721411408772

50. Bengtson, V. L., Gans, D., Putney, N. M., & Silverstein, M. (2009). *Handbook of Theories on Aging* Vol.2

51. Parasuraman, A., Zeithaml, V. A., & Berry, L. L. (1998). "Alternative scales for measuring service quality: a comparative assessment based on psychometric and diagnostic criteria." *Handbuch Dienstleistungsmanagement.* Springer:449-482.

52. Gazzaley, A., & Nobre, A. C. (2012). "Top-down modulation: bridging selective attention and working memory". *Trends Cogn Sci*, 16(2): 129-135. doi:10.1016/j.tics.2011.11.014

53. Attention processes involve almost all brain structures, including the striated cortex, the prestriate cortex, the medial temporal cortex, the inferior parietal cortex, the frontal eye fields, the prefrontal cortex, the cingulate gyrus, the nucleus pulvinaris, the nucleus lateral geniculate, the substantia nigra, and the superior colliculus..

54. Leclercq, M., & Zimmermann, P. (2004). *Applied neuropsychology of attention: theory, diagnosis and rehabilitation.* Psychology Press.

55. Gazzaley, A., & Nobre, A. C. (2012). "Top-down modulation: bridging selective attention and working memory". *Trends Cogn Sci*, 16(2): 129-135. doi:10.1016/j.tics.2011.11.014

56. Bengtson, M., Martin, R., Sawrie, S., Gilliam, F., Faught, E., Morawetz, R., & Kuzniecky, R. (2000). "Gender, Memory, and Hippocampal Volumes: Relationships in Temporal Lobe Epilepsy". *Epilepsy Behav,* 1(2): 112-119. doi:10.1006/ebeh.2000.0051

57. Yinger, O. S., & Cevasco, A. (2014). "Understanding neuroscience within the field of medical music therapy" en *Medical Music Therapy: Building a comprehensive program.* Silver Spring, MD: American Music Therapy Association.

58. Gardner, H. (1985). *The Mind's New Science: A History of the Cognitive Revolution.* New York: Basic Books.

59. Fodor, J. (1983). *The Modularity of Mind.* MIT Press.
60. Pinker, S. (2009). *How the Mind Works.* New York: Norton.

61. van der Schyff, Dylan. (2013). "Music, Meaning and the Embodied Mind: Towards an Enactive Approach to Music Cognition". MA Diss. University of Sheffield.

62. Changizi, M. (2011). *Harnessed: How language and Music Mimicked Nature and Transformed Ape Into Man.* Dallas: BenBella.

63. Tomasello, M. (1999). *The Cultural Origins of Human Cognition.* Cambridge, MA: Harvard UP.

64. Kempler, D. (2005). *Neurocognitive disorders in aging*: Sage.

65. Pascual-Leone, A., & Hamilton, R. (2001). "The metamodal organization of the brain". *Progress in brain research,* 134: 427-445.

66. Small, C. (1999). *Musicking: The Meaning of Performing and Listening.* Middletown, CT: Wesleyan UP.

67. Blacking, J. (1976). *How Musical is Man?.* London: Faber.

68. Korom, Frank J. (2006). *Village of Painters: Narrative Scrolls from West Bengal.* Santa Fe: Museum of New Mexico Press.

69. Andy Clark & David Chalmers. (2008). "The extended mind" en *Analysis,* 58(1), 7-19.

70. James Gibson. (1966). *The Senses Considered as Perceptual Systems.* Boston: Houghton-Miffflin.

71. Campbell, M. R. (1991). "Musical learning and the development of psychological processes in perception and cognition". *Bulletin of the Council for Research in Music Education:* 35-48.

72. Ortman, J. M., Velkoff, V. A., & Hogan, H. (2014). "An aging nation: the older population in the United States". United States Census Bureau, Economics and Statistics Administration, US Department of Commerce.

73. Kramer, A. F., Humphrey, D. G., Larish, J. F., Logan, G. D., & Strayer, D. L. (1994). "Aging and inhibition: beyond a unitary view of inhibitory processing in attention". *Psychol Aging*, 9(4), 491-512.

74. Hall, C. B., Lipton, R. B., Sliwinski, M., Katz, M. J., Derby, C. A., & Verghese, J. (2009). "Cognitive activities delay onset of memory decline in persons who develop dementia". *Neurology*, 73(5), 356-361. doi:10.1212/WNL.0b013e3181b04ae3.

75. Rodrigues, A. C., Loureiro, M. A., & Caramelli, P. (2013). "Long-term musical training may improve different forms of visual attention ability". *Brain Cogn*, 82(3), 229-235. doi:10.1016/j.bandc.2013.04.009

76. Lehmann, A. C., & Davidson, J. W. (2002). "Taking an acquired skills perspective on music performance." *The new handbook of research on music teaching and learning*, 2, 542- 560.

78. Grant, M. D., & Brody, J. A. (2004). "Musical experience and dementia. Hypothesis". *Aging Clin Exp Res*, 16(5), 403-405.

78. Gaser, C. and G. Schlaug (2003). "Brain structures differ between musicians and nonmusicians." J. *Neurosci.* 23(27): 9240-9245.

79. Schlaug, G. (2001). "The brain of musicians. A model for functional and structural adaptation." Ann. N. Y. *Acad. Sci.* 930: 281-299.

80. Wan, C. Y., & Schlaug, G. (2010). "Music making as a tool for promoting brain plasticity across the life span". *Neuroscientist*, 16(5), 566-577. doi:10.1177/1073858410377805

81. Gaser, C., & Schlaug, G. (2003). "Brain structures differ between musicians and nonmusicians", *JNeurosci*, 23(27), 9240-9245.

82.Schulz, M., Ross, B., & Pantev, C. (2003). "Evidence for training-induced crossmodal reorganization of cortical functions in trumpet players". *Neuroreport,* 14(1), 157-161. doi:10.1097/01.wnr.0000053061.10406.c7

83. Kraus, N., & Chandrasekaran, B. (2010). "Music training for the development of auditory skills". *Nat Rev Neurosci,* 11(8), 599-605. doi:10.1038/nrn2882.

84. Bever T.& Chiarello, R. (2009) "Cerebral dominance in musicians and nonmusicians". *The Journal of Neuropsychiatry and Clinical Neurosciences.* Winter; 21 (1) :94-7.

85. Habibi, A.(2011). "Cortical activity during music perception; comparing musicians and non-musicians". Ph.D. Diss. University of California Irvine.

86. Skoe, E. and N. Kraus (2010). "Auditory brain stem response to complex sounds: a tutorial." *Ear Hear.* 31(3): 302-324.

87. Percaccio CR, Pruette AL, Mistry ST, Chen YH, Kilgard MP. (2007) "Sensory experience determines enrichment-induced plasticity in rat auditory cortex". *Brain Res.* 2007 Oct 12;1174:76-91. doi: 10.1016/j.brainres.2007.07.062. Epub 2007 Aug 9. PMID: 17854780.

88. Kraus, N. and B. Chandrasekaran (2010). "Music training for the development of auditory skills." *Nature Reviews Neuroscience* 11(8): 599-605.

89 Keverne, E. B. (2004). Understanding well-being in the evolutionary context of brain development. *Proceedings of the Royal Society of London,* 359: 1349–1358.

90. Krizman, J., J. Slater, E. Skoe, V. Marian and N. Kraus (2015). "Neural processing of speech in children is influenced by extent of bilingual experience." *Neurosci. Lett.* 585: 48-53.

91. Vuust, P., E. Brattico, M. Seppänen, R. Näätänen and M. Tervaniemi (2012). "Practiced musical style shapes auditory skills." *Ann. N. Y. Acad. Sci.* 1252(1): 139-146.

92. "Neurotransmitter," in *The Columbia Encyclopedia,* New York: Columbia University Press, 2013, consultada December 17, 2014, http://literati.credoreference.com.

93. Anthony L. Vaccarino and Abba J. Kastin, "Endogenous Opiates: 2000," *Peptides 22* (2001): 2257.

94. Berger,M. Gray, J.A. and Roth, B. (2009). "The Expanded Biology of Serotonin," *Annual Review of Medicine* 60 : 356.

95. Nakajima, S. et al. (2013) "The Potential Role of Dopamine D3 Receptor Neurotransmission in Cognition," *European Neuropsychopharmacology* 23, no. 8 : 800-1.

96. Falk, D. (1983). "Cerebral cortices of east African early hominids". *Science,* 221: 1072–1074.

97. Saarikallio, S., and Erkkilä, J. (2007). "The role of music in adolescents' mood regulation". *Psychology of Music,* 35(1), 88-109. Doi: 10.1177/0305735607068889.

98. Schäfer, T., Smukalla, M., and Oelker, S-A. (2014). "How music changes our lives: A qualitative study of the long-term effects of intense emotional experiences". *Psychology of Music,* 42(4), 525-544. Doi: 10.1177/0305735613482024.

99. Trainor, L. J., Tsang, C. D., & Cheung, V. H. W. (2002). "Preference for Sensory Consonance in 2- and 4-month-old Infants". *Music Perception,* 20: 187-194.

100.Cummingham, J., Sterling, R. (1988). "Developmental Change in the Understanding of Affective Meaning in Music". *Motivation and Emotion,* 12: 399-413.

101. Izard, C. (1977). *Human emotions.* New York, NY: Plenum Press.

102. Ekman, P. (1999). "Basic emotions". In T. Dalgleish and M. Power (Eds.), *Handbook of cognition and emotion.* New York, NY: John Wiley and Sons Ltd.:45-60.

103.Barrett, L. (2006a). "Are emotions natural kinds?". *Perspectives on Psychological Science,* 1(1), 28-58. Doi: 10.1111/j.1745-6916.2006.00003.x.

104. Russell, J. (2003). "Core affect and the psychological construction of emotion". *Psychological Review*, 110(1), 145-172. Doi: 10.1037/0033-295X.110.1.145.

105. Scherer, K., Schorr, A., and Johnstone, T. (2001). *Appraisal processes in emotion: Theory, methods, research.* New York, NY: Oxford University Press.

106. Ekman, P., and Cortado, D. (2011). "What is meant by calling emotions basic?". *Emotion Review*, 3(4), 364-370. Doi: 10.1177/1754073911410740.

107. Darwin, C. (1872). *The expression of emotions in man and animals.* London, UK: John Murray.

108. Izard, C. (2007). "Basic emotions, natural kinds, emotion schemas, and a new paradigm". *Perspectives on Psychological Science*, 2(3), 260-280. Doi:10.1111/ j.1745-6916.2007.00044.x.

109. Ekman, P., and Cortado, D. (2011). "What is meant by calling emotions basic?". *Emotion Review*, 3(4), 364-370. Doi: 10.1177/1754073911410740.

110. Kreibig, S. (2010). "Autonomic nervous system activity in emotion: A review". *Biological Psychology*, 84(3), 394-421. Doi: 10.1016/j.biopsycho.2010.03.010.

111. LeDoux, J. (2003). "The emotional brain, fear, and the amygdala". Cellular and *Molecular Neurobiology*, 23(4-5), 727-738. Doi: doi.org/10.1023/A:1025048802629.

112. Peretz, G., N I., Johnsen, E., and Adolphs, R. (2007). "Amygdala damage impairs emotion recognition from music". *Neuropsychologica*, 45(2), 236-244. Doi:10.1016/ j.neuropsychologia.2006.07.012.

113. Bannister, S. Craig (2020). "A Framework of Distinct Musical Chills: Theoretical, Causal, and Conceptual Evidence", Durham theses, Durham University. Available at Durham E-Theses Online: http://etheses.dur.ac. uk/13582 /

114. Tomkins, S. (1984). "Affect theory". In K. Scherer and P. Ekman (Eds.), *Approaches to emotion*. Hillsdale, NJ: Erlbaum:163-195.

115. Scherer, K., and Coutinho, E. (2013). "How music creates emotion: A multifactorial process approach". In T. Cochrane, B. Fantini, and K. Scherer (Eds.), *The emotional power of music: Multidisciplinary perspectives on musical arousal, expression, and social control*. New York, NY: Oxford University Press:121-145.

116. Gross, J., and Barrett, L. F. (2011). "Emotion generation and emotion regulation: One or two depends on your point of view". *Emotion Review*, 3(1), 8-16. Doi:10.1177/1754073910380974.

117. Darwin, C. (1902). *The Descent of Man and Selection in Relation to Sex, part II*. New York: P.F. Collier & Son.

118. Juslin, P., Vastfjall, D. 2008. "Emotional Responses to Music: The Need to Consider Underlying Mechanism". *Behavioral Brain Sciences*, 31: 559-621.

119. Zentner, M. Grandjean, D., K. Scherer. (2008). "Emotions Evoked by the Sound of Music: Characterization, Classification, and Measurement". *Emotion*, 8(4): 494-521.

120. IBID.

121. Papp, G., Kovac, S., Frese, A., & Evers, S. (2014). "The impact of temporal lobe epilepsy on musical ability". *Seizure*, 23, 533–536.

122. Sloboda, J. (1991). "Music Structure and Emotional Response: Some Empirical Findings". *Psychology of Music*, 19: 110-120.

123. Kringelbach, M. L., & Berridge, K. C. (Eds.). (2010). *The pleasures of the brain*. New York:Oxford University Press.

124. Kringelbach, M. L., & Berridge, K. C. (2010). "The Neuroscience of Happiness and Pleasure". *Social Research: An International Quarterly*, Volume 77, Number 2, Summer. 659-678.

125. Becker, S., Bräscher, A-K., Bannister, S., Bensafi, M., Calma-Birling, D., Chan, R., Wang, Y. (2019). "The role of hedonics in the human affectome". *Neuroscience and Biobehavioural Reviews*, 102, 221-241. Doi: 10.1016/j.neubiorev.2019.05.003.

126. Liu, X., Hairston, J., Schrier, M., and Fan, J. (2011). "Common and distinct networks underlying reward valence and processing stages: A meta-analysis of functional neuroimaging studies". Neuroscience and Biobehavioural Reviews, 35(5), 1219-1236. Doi: 10.1016/j.neubiorev.2010.12.012.

127. La anhedonia, proveniente del griego hedoné que significa placer, es la incapacidad para experimentar placer.

128. Mas-Herrero, E., Zatorre, R. J., Rodriguez-Fornells, A., & Marco-Pallarés, J. (2014). "Dissociation between Musical and Monetary Reward Responses in Specific Musical Anhedonia." *Current Biology*, 24, 1–6.

129. Csikszentmihalyi, M. (1990). *Flow: The Psychology of Optimal Experience; Steps Toward Enhancing the Quality of Life*. New York: HarperPerennial.

130. NIMH (2016). Mission. Obtenido en: https://www.nih.gov/about-nih/what-we-do/nihalmanac/national-institute-mental-health-nimh.

131. Ch. Wickramarathne, J. Chun Phuoc, J. Tham. (2020). "The impact of wellness dimensions on the academic performance of undergraduates of Government universities in Sri Lanka". European Journal of Public Health Studies. Scientific Figure on ResearchGate. https://www.researchgate.net/figure/Six-dimensions-of-wellness-model-Source-Hettler-1977_fig1_342769817 [consultado 23 Aug, 2020]

132. Hettler, B. (1977). *Six Dimension Model*. Stevens Point, WI: National Wellness Institute.

133. Hutchison, B. (2016). "The Role of Music Among Healthy Older Performance Musicians". North Dakota State University. Doctoral Diss.

134. Chanda, M. L., & Levitin, D. J. (2013). "The neurochemistry of music". *Trends in Cognitive Sciences*, 17(4), 179-193. DOI 10.1016/j.tics.2013.02.007.

135. Keeler Jason, Roth Edward, Neuser Brittany, Spitsbergen John, Waters Daniel, Vianney John-Mary. (2015)."The neurochemistry and social flow of singing: bonding and oxytocin". *Frontiers in Human Neuroscience*, V. 9 , 518. Online: https://www.frontiersin.org/article/10.3389/fnhum.2015.00518

136. Lori A. Custodero. (2012). "The Call to Create: Flow Experience in Music Learning and Teaching", David Hargreaves, Dorothy Miell and Raymond MacDonald (eds.), *Musical Imaginations: Multidisciplinary Perspectives on Creativity, Performance and Perception*. Oxford: Oxford University Press, 369-84.

137.The five musical rights include the right of all children and adults to express themselves freely through music, the right to learn musical languages and skills, the right to interact with music through direct participation, appreciation, creation, and access to information. The right of all musicians to develop their careers and to disseminate their artistic work through all available media and the right to obtain recognition and fair compensation for their work. https://www.imc-cim.org/about-imc-separator/five-music-rights.html

138. Three initiates, (2009). *The Kybalion: A Study of the Hermetic Philosophy of Ancient Egypt*. Mineola,New York: Dover Publications Inc.

139. Conrad-Da'oud, E. (2012). *Life on Land: The Story of Continuum, the World-Renowned Self-Discovery and Movement Method*. North Atlantic Books, Berkeley.

140. Schroeder, D. Poeppel and E. Zion Golumbic (2017). "Neural Entrainment to the Beat: The "Missing-Pulse" Phenomenon" en *Journal of Neuroscience* 28 June, 2017, 37 (26) 6331-6341; DOI: https://doi.org/10.1523/JNEUROSCI.2500-16.2017

141. I. Tal, Large,E. W., Rabinovitch, E., Wei, Y., Schroeder, Ch. E., Poeppel, D. and Zion Golumbic, E. (2017). "Neural Entrainment to the Beat: The "Missing-Pulse" Phenomenon" en *Journal of Neuroscience* 28 June, 2017, 37 (26) 6331-6341; DOI: https://doi.org/10.1523/ JNEUROSCI.2500-16.2017.

142. Arcangeli A. (2000). "Dance and Health: The Renaissance Physicians". Dance Research: *The Journal of the Society for Dance Research*, Vol. 18, No. 1. Published by: Edinburgh University Press. Edimburgh. 3-30.

143. Paul Krack, "Relicts of Dancing Mania: The Dancing Procession of Echternach," *Neurology* 53, no. 9 (1999): 2169-72.

144. Bicais, M. (1669). "La manire de regler la sante par ce qui nous environne, par ce que nous recevons, et par les exercices, ou par la gymnastique moderne" (Aix: chez Charles David, 1669), pp. 280-8.

145. Shaffer, J. (2012). "Neuroplasticity and positive psychology in clinical practice: A review for combined benefits psychology." *PSYCH*, 3(12A), 1110-1115. doi: 10.4236/ psych.2012.312A164.

146. Eriksson, P. S., Perfilieva, E., Björk-Eriksson, T., Alborn, A. M., Nordborg, C., Peterson, D. A., & Gage, F. H. (1998). "Neurogenesis in the adult human hippocampus". *Nature medicine*, 4(11), 1313-1317.

147. Kempermann, G., Gast, D., & Gage, F. H. (2002). "Neuroplasticity in old age: Sustained fivefold induction of hippocampal neurogenesis by long term environmental enrichment". *Annals of Neurology*, 52(2), 135-143.

148. Lynn-Seraphine, P. (2016). "Neurodrumming: Towards an integral mental fitness training for healthy aging". Diss. Master Psychology, California State University, Irvine.

149. Geiser, E. Zähle, T., Jacke, L. & Meyer, M. (2008). "The neural correlate of speech rhythm as evidenced by metrical speech processing." *Journal of Cognitive Neuroscience*, 20(3), 541-552. doi:10.1162/jocn.2008.20029.

150. Dale, J.A., Hyatt, J., Hollerman, J. (2007). "The Neuroscience of Dance and the Dance of Neuroscience: Defining a Path of Inquiry". *The Journal of Aesthetic Education*, Volume 41, Number 3, Fall 2007. 89-110.

151. Stobart, H. & Cross, I. (2000). "The Andean anacrusis? Rhythmic structure and perception in Easter songs of northern Potosi, Bolivia." *British Journal of Ethnomusicology, 9(2), 63-94.*

152. Kalender, B. Trehub, S.E., & Schellenberg, E.G. (2012). "Cross-cultural differences in meter perception". *Psychological Research*, 77(2), 196-203. Doi:10.1007/s00426-012-0427-y

153. Hannon, E.E., & Trehub, S.E. (2005b). "Tuning in to musical rhythms: infants learn more readily than adults." *Proceedings of the National Academy of Sciences of the United States of America*, 102 (35), 12639-12643. Doi:10.1073/pnas.0504254102

154. Witek MAG, Clarke EF, Wallentin M, Kringelbach ML, Vuust P (2014) "Syncopation, Body-Movement and Pleasure" in *Groove Music*. PLoS ONE 9(4): e94446. doi:10.1371/journal.pone.0094446

155. Davies, J., & McVicar, A. (2000). "Issues in effective pain control". 1: Assessment and education. *International Journal of Palliative Nursing*, 6(2), 58-65.

156. Allen, J. (2013a). "Pain management with adults". In J. Allen (Ed.), *Guidelines for music therapy practice in adult medical care* (pp. 35-61). University Park, IL: Barcelona Publishers.

157. Dileo, C. (1999). *Music therapy and medicine: Theoretical and clinical applications.* Silver Spring, MD: American Music Therapy Association.

158. Bradt, J., Dileo, C., & Potvin, N. (2013). "Music for stress and anxiety reduction in coronary heart disease patients." *The Cochrane Database of Systematic Reviews,* 12, CD006577

159. Gatchel, R. J., Peng, Y. B., Peters, M. L., Fuchs, P. N., & Turk, D. C. (2007). "The biopsychosocial approach to chronic pain: Scientific advances and future directions". *Psychological Bulletin,* 133(4), 581-624.

160. Melzack, R. (2010). Pain theories. In I. B. Weiner, & W. E. Craighead (Eds.), The corsini encyclopedia of psychology (4th ed.,). Hoboken, NJ: John Wiley & Sons, Inc. doi:10.1002/9780470479216.corpsy0630

161. Melzack, R. (1999). "From the gate to the neuromatrix". *Pain,* Suppl 6, S121-S126. doi:10.1016/S0304-3959(99)00145-1

162. Bardia, A., Barton, D. L., Prokop, L. J., Bauer, B. A., & Moynihan, T. J. (2006). "Efficacy of complementary and alternative medicine therapies in relieving cancer pain: A systematic review". *Journal of Clinical Oncology,* 24(34), 5457-5464.

163. Gallagher, L. M., Lagman, R., Walsh, D., Davis, M. P., & LeGrand, S. B. (2006). "The clinical effects of music therapy in palliative medicine". *Supportive Care in Cancer,* 14, 859- 866.

164. Hilliard, R. (2003). "The effects of music therapy on the quality and length of life of people diagnosed with terminal cancer." Journal *of Music Therapy,* 40, 113-137.

165. Ferrer, A. J. (2007). "The effect of live music on decreasing anxiety in patients undergoing chemotherapy treatment". *Journal of Music Therapy,* 44, 242-255.

166. Clark, M., Isaacks-Downton, G., Wells, N., Redlin-Frazier, S., Eck, C., Hepworth, J. T., & Chakravarthy, B. (2006). "Use of preferred music to reduce emotional distress and symptom activity during radiation therapy." *Journal of Music Therapy,* 43, 247-265.

167. Sahler, O. J. Z., Hunter, B. C., Liesveld, J. L. (2003). "The effect of using music therapy with relaxation imagery in the management of patients undergoing bone marrow transplantation: A pilot feasibility study." *Alternative Therapies in Health and Medicine,* 9(6), 70-74.

168. Edward, J (1998). "Music Therapy for children with severe burn injury." *Music Therapy Perspectives,* 16: 21-26.

169. Zimmerman, I., Nieveen, J., Barnason, S. & Schamaderer, M. (1996)."The effects of music intervention is postoperative pain and sleep in coronary artery bypass graft (CRGB) patients". *Scholarly Inquiry for Nursing Practice: An International Journal,* 10. 153-170.

170. Galpin, W. (1937) *The Music of the Sumerians: And their Immediate Successors, the Babylonians and Assyrians.* Cambridge University Press.

171. Meyer-Baer, K. (2015). *Music of the Spheres and the Dance of Death.* Princeton University Press. 224-241.

172.Qi Kun (2014). "Sonic expressions of cosmological awareness: a comparative study of funeral rituals among Han Chinese living in the Yangzi River Valley". Yearbook for Traditional Music Vol. 46. Cambridge University Press :159-169.

173. Coclanis, A., Coclanis P. (2005). "Jazz Funeral: A Living Tradition". *Southern Cultures,* Volume 11, Number 2. The University of North Carolina Press. 86-92.

174. Austin, D. (2009). *The Theory and Practice of Vocal Psychotherapy: Songs of the self.* London: Jessica Kingsley Publishers.

175. https://chaliceofrepose.org/

176. Cooper, L. "Your Healing Voice - The benefits of singing for health and wellbeing" en https://www.britishacademyofsoundtherapy.com/wp-content/uploads/2020/07/Your-Healing-Voice-Article-sing-for-health-research-3.pdf

177. The Oxford Happiness Questionnaire http://www.blake-group.com/sites/default/files/ assessments/ Oxford_Happiness_Questionnaire.pdf

178. Bart de Boer (2017). "Evolution of speech and evolution of language". Published online: 3 August 2016, Psychonomic Society, Inc. 2016 Psychon Bull Rev (2017) 24:158–162 DOI 10.3758/s13423-016-1130-6.

179. Darwin, C. (1872/1998). The Expression of the Emotions in Man and Animals. Oxford: Oxford University Press.

180. Kelley, D. B. (2004). "Vocal communication in frogs". Current Opinion in *Neurobiology*, 14: 751–757.

181. Insel, T. R. (2010). "The challenge of translation in social neuroscience: A review of oxytocin, vasopressin, and affiliative behavior". *Neuron*, 65: 768–779.

182. Kanwal, J. S., and Ehret, G. (2006). *Behavior and Neurodynamics for Auditory Communication.* Cambridge: Cambridge University Press.

183. Sterne, J. (2003). *The Audible Past: Cultural Origins of Sound Reproduction.* Durham: Duke University Press.15.

184. IBID, 54.

185. Auenbrugger, L. (1936). "On the Percussion of the Chest" Translated by John Forbes. *Bulletin of the History of Medicine* 4. Cit. Sterne, J. (2003).

186. Laennec, R.T.H.A. (1830) *Treatise on the Diseases of the Chest and on Mediate Auscultation.* 3 ed. Translated by John Forbes. New York: Samuel Wood; Collins and Hannay. Cit. Sterne, J. (2003).

187. Arozqueta, C. (2018). "Heartbeats and the Arts: A Historical Connection". *Leonardo* 51 (1): 33–39. doi: https://doi.org/10.1162/LEON_a_01152

188. http://musicwithmachines.org/hco/

189. Sweeley, C.C., Holland, J.F, Towson, D.S., Chamberlin, B.A. (1987) "Interactive and Multi-Sensory Analysis of Complex Mixtures by an Automated Gas Chromatography System," Journal of Chromatography 399: 173–181.

190. Ohno, S. y Ohno, M. (1986) "The All Pervasive Principle of Repetitious Recurrence Governs Not Only Coding Sequence Construction but Also Human Endeavor in Musical Composition," *Immunogenetics* 24: 71–78.

191. Ohno, S. (1993) "A Song in Praise of Peptide Palindromes," *Leukemia* 7 Supp. 2 S157–S159.

192. Morey, L.W. (1989) "Musings on Biomuse," Science News 135: 307.

193. Han, Y.C., & Han, B. (2014). Skin Pattern Sonification as a New Timbral Expression. Leonardo Music Journal 24(1), 41-43. https://www.muse.jhu.edu/article/561861.

194. IBID.

195. Pelling AE, Sehati S, Gralla EB, Valentine JS, Gimzewski JK. (2004). "Local nanomechanical motion of the cell wall of Saccharomyces cerevisiae", Science. 2004 Aug 20;305 (5687):1147-50.

196. Gadamer, Hans-Georg. (1989). *Truth and Method.* 2nd ed. Translated by W. Glen-Doepel, translation revised by Joel Weinsheimer and Donald G. Marshall. London: Continuum. First published 1960 as Wahrheit und Methode: Grundzüge einer philosophischen Hermeneutik (Tübingen: Mohr). 2nd ed. of translation first published 1989 (London: Sheed and Ward): 355.

197. Dacey, J. (1999). *Concepts of creativity: A history.* In M. A. Runco & S.R. Pritzer (Eds), Encyclopedia of creativity, Vol.1 A–H. San Diego, CA: Academic Press.

198. Albert, R. S., & Runco, M. A. (1999). "The history of creativity research". In R. S. Sternberg (Ed.), *Handbook of human creativity.* New York, NY: Cambridge University Press: 16–31

199. Vartanian, O., et al. *Neuroscience of Creativity*. The MIT Press, 2013. Project MUSE. muse.jhu.edu/book/46971.

200. Roe BE, Tilley MR, Gu HH, Beversdorf DQ, Sadee W, Haab TC, et al. (2009) "Financial and Psychological Risk Attitudes Associated with Two Single Nucleotide Polymorphisms in the Nicotine Receptor (CHRNA4) Gene". PLoS ONE 4(8): e6704. https://doi.org/10.1371/journal.pone.0006704.

201. Zuckerman , M. (1994). *Behavioral expressions and bio-social expressions of sensation seeking* . Cambridge : Cambridge University Press.

202. Miller, G. F. (2001). "Aesthetic Fitness: How Sexual Selection Shaped Artistic Virtuosity as a Fitness Indicator and Aesthetic Preferences as Mate Choice Criteria". *Bulletin of Psychology and the Arts*, 2, 20-25.

203. Hinde, R. A. & Fisher, J. (1951). Further observations on the opening of milk bottles by birds. *British Birds*,44, 393-396.

204. Wallas, G. (1926). *Art of thought*. New York, NY: Harcourt Brace.

205. http://www.furious.com/perfect/stockhauseninterview.html

206. Lapidaki, E. (2007). "Learning from Masters of Music Creativity: Shaping Compositional Experiences in Music Education." *Philosophy of Music Education Review*, 15(2): 93-117. Revisado May 20, 2021 en http://www.jstor.org/stable/40327276.

207. P.A. Schilpp, ed., (1959). *Albert Einstein: Philosopher-Scientist*. New York: Harpers,Vol. : 2:45.

208. http://www.personal.psu.edu/faculty/m/e/meb26/INART55/varese.html

209. Eidsheim N. S. (2015). *Sensing sound. singing & listening as vibrational practice*. Durham, London: Duke University Press: 16.

210. Huang J., Gamble D., Sarnlertsophon K., Wang X., Hsiao S. (2012). *Feeling music: integration of auditory and tactile inputs in musical meter perception.* PLoS One 7:e48496.

211. Root-Bernstein, R.S. (2001). "Music, Creativity and Scientific Thinking". *Leonardo* 34(1), 63-68. https://www.muse.jhu.edu/article/19631.

212. IBID.

213. The Group pof Five was a grup of prominent nationalistic Russian composers formed by Mili Balákirev (el líder), César Cuí, Modest Músorgski, Nikolái Rimski-Kórsakov y Aleksandr Borodín.

214. Root-Bernstein, R.S. (2001). "Music, Creativity and Scientific Thinking." *Leonardo* 34(1): 63-68. https://www.muse.jhu.edu/article/19631.

215. Milgram, R., Dunn, R. y Price, G.E. eds., "Teaching and Counseling Gifted and Talented Adolescents: An International Learning Style Perspective". New York: Praeger.

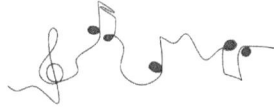

ABOUT THE AUTHOR

Patricia Caicedo is a soprano, musicologist and physician whose scholarship and performances center Latin American and Iberian art song. She has released eleven albums and published numerous scholarly editions of scores and books, including *The Latin American Art Song: Sounds of the Imagined Nations*, the go-to history on its subject.

She is also an avid performer of these works, having performed at important halls in Europe and the Americas in addition to founding and directing the *Barcelona Festival of Song*, which focuses on the performance and study of Latin American and Iberian art songs in Spanish, Catalan, and Portuguese.

She is the host of the podcast, *Latin American and Iberian Art Song,* in which she interviews composers and leading experts from across the world.

Patricia holds a Ph.D. in musicology from the Universidad Complutense de Madrid and a Medical Doctor's degree from the Escuela Colombiana de Medicina. She is an Executive Board Member of the International Music Council a UNESCO partner organization.

PATRICIACAICEDO.COM

Follow Patricia Caicedo on social **media,** communicate with her, listen to her music and podcast, invite her to speak at your institution, ask her questions or simply share your ideas about the book

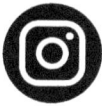

@patriciacaicedobcn

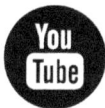

https://spoti.fi/2XQwHHS

Twitter @PatriciaCaicedo

youtube.com/singerpat

Facebook /FansPatriciaCaicedo

Linkedin /in/patriciacaicedo

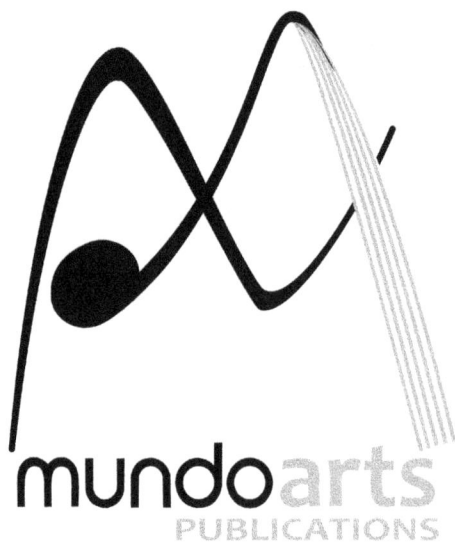

mundoarts
PUBLICATIONS

www.mundoarts.com

www.ingramcontent.com/pod-product-compliance
Lightning Source LLC
Chambersburg PA
CBHW051728260326
41914CB00040B/2015/J